Brave Will

Brave Will: Love Letters from a Father to His Son

Copyright 2009 Matthew Hladun
All rights reserved. Published 2009.
Printed in the United States of America

ISBN 978-0-557-27474-1

For more information visit: www.bravewill.org

*"Strength does not come from physical capacity.
It comes from an indomitable will."*

Mahatma Gandhi

Foreword

There are times in our lives that we are going along thinking about mundane things in life. We may even be taking for granted the routine habits we do each day. We enjoy the wonders of new excitement we hear about on some days and on others just enjoy the routine.

Many months ago I found out about an impending event that would bring about great change in my life and many other lives around the world. It all started as one of those normal joys we hear about that grew into an incredible journey. I have a group of friends that are as dear to me as those that I have close to me at my home. This particular group of friends was all brought about via a chat room on the Oprah.com website. We each had reasons to one by one come to this site to find what turned out to be life altering love and support. This group of woman all over the age of sixty found day by day a growing relationship that has transcended the miles that separate us.

We started talking in the chat room and evolved to an email group of a dozen women. We share all the many things that happen in our daily lives and reach out to one another in the midst of every life event that comes our way.

One of those events was when one of our groups' members was all excited about the impending birth of a new grandchild. This grandchild was going to be the third child of her son and daughter-in-law. They were selling their home and planning on building a new one. We all rejoiced when we found that their home sold quickly. That was good news even though a very pregnant mom was going to need to live somewhere while waiting for this great impending birth. Arrangements were made to share the time between both sets of grandparents home till this precious gift was to be born.

We all would hear day by day the progress of the pregnancy and of the new house to be built. There were so many details of storing household belongings, moving with two young boys into the warm home of first paternal grandparents then to maternal grandparents.

The time was approaching for this little boy to be born. We all celebrated the fact that two brothers were about to add a third boy to this family. I remember loving all the post about this cute family. I also remember perhaps taking for granted the full impact of this family and how the future was going to bring us all on a road none of us could have ever dreamed. The little boy would have a name that was about to be etched into the brains of people around the world, not just our dozen women. This little boy would be known as Will.

The child was born and all was going beautifully. We all could be excited over pictures and a young family preparing for a new home and all the promise that youth brings to a growing family. The two brothers, Ben and Max, were so excited about the new brother and plans were being made daily. Life for this family was going at a rapid pace and not one of us suspected, most of all Will's family, the impending danger lurking near.

There came a time when little Will wasn't even quite eight weeks old when a very alert mom noticed something not quite right. She noticed that when changing a diaper that Will seemed to be very uncomfortable and had a swelling in his leg that she knew wasn't normal. Will was taken to his doctor to have his leg checked out. In the ensuing time it was found that this child had a serious problem that was about to change the destiny of this family, all their friends, our "O" group, and eventually the world. Will was found to have what every parent fears most: An illness that was about to turn their lives upside down.

The horrible word came that Will had a tumor in his right leg and one in his brain. The tumors were malignant and the prognosis was grave. This incredible family had to face the horror of making decisions each day that seemed impossible to fathom for any parent.

This is where the miracle of this story begins to unfold. Will was not given much time on this earth per his doctors. The family had to try to comprehend the unbelievable news of a baby only 8 weeks old who had terminal cancer. My God in Heaven how could this be? He was given only a short time to live. Will and God had other plans. The miracle of this story was that Will was going to become Brave Will and he, in his short life, was going to show doctors he could beat odds that were stacked against him. He would go through painful chemo therapy that would bring with it so many horrible complications and bounce back each time.

At one point the doctors were able to come in with the unbelievable news that the lesion in his brain was no longer showing. We all praised God for this miracle. Will would continue additional rounds of chemo therapy to continue to remove all cancer cells in his body. The brain lesions continued to remain gone but the tumor in his leg remained and would not go away.

Will would have many complications and bounce back from each one. Will even began to take little trips out of the hospital to be with his family in nearby hotel where they stayed near the hospital while he endured all the treatment. Will's family would learn as we all would that this little boy was not your average boy. This boy was not only brave but a fighter like no one had ever seen. This little baby was busy teaching his family and the world about what fighting means. The story progressed and hope was strong for all who knew about this story. Then the terrible news came that the tumor in his leg had grown at such a rapid rate it had broken his femur and spread the cancer cells to his entire body. There had been a surgery planned to remove Will's right leg but that was cancelled for the prognosis was grave. Now all that could be done was keep Brave Will comfortable. The heartbreak within the family is unthinkable yet each of us is with this family to the deepest part of our faith and love.

What is the impact of all of this on our lives? The impact is that a little baby was born with the same promise of each child created. We watched as God touched this child from birth, illness, to glory that will be Brave Will's. We can see that as God loves this child he loves each of us with the same unlimited devotion. Brave Will may only have had a short time on earth but he just kept teaching about ability to fight against insurmountable odds. Brave Will was blessed with parents that have allowed us to join in this journey with them through an almost daily journal entry written by Will's father, Matt. I know God chose this child to have these parents while at the same time chose each of us on this journey to share in the faith of a young father, mother, brothers, grandparents, and a world of those who believe. Angels whisper into the ear of this baby the answers we all seek. Will is going to know all the answers before those of us who have been on the planet longer, and that is alright. God is in His Heaven and I have been lucky enough to learn hope never gives up. Faith believes in the unseen and each of our spiritual lives has grown in abundance because of faith.

Nancy Ratcliff-Rondeau

Letters to Will

The letters on the following pages were originally posted on a website from September 17, 2008 through February 6, 2009

WEDNESDAY, SEPTEMBER 17, 2008

I've thought a lot about how I wanted to approach using this site. When I was an English teacher, I used to tell my students, "Know your audience before you start writing". This task will be more difficult for me because I don't know who the audience will be--family, friends, colleagues, strangers...

I decided to approach this in a different way and have my audience be the one who I really want to hear my words, my son Will. I'm hoping one day, Will can look back on what Tammy and I wrote and know how much we fought with him and cried for him. I suspect what gets written in the days to come will be therapeutic for Tammy and me, but at the same time, I have difficulty coming to grips with the fact that I am writing this at all. So stay with us through this difficult journey and keep us in your thoughts whenever you can.

WEDNESDAY, SEPTEMBER 17, 2008

Brave Will,

I apologize right away--despite being a little more on the quiet side when speaking, I do tend to be long-winded when I write. I imagine you at fifteen, looking back at my words and thinking, "Geez dad, do I have to read all of this?"

I guess I'll start by explaining how we all got to this point. You were born on July 14, 2008 and weighed a healthy eight pounds. You gave your mom a difficult time when she was pregnant, and we were just thankful that you fought with her for nine months to come out as beautiful as you did. Though, like your two older brothers, you looked nothing like me! Your birth and first two months of life were as normal as what your mom and I experienced with Ben and Max. You cried when you were hungry, slept when you were tired, and were a typical baby. Somewhere during the month of September, we noticed that you didn't like to have your diaper changed--your mom was thankful because she thought you just didn't like to be nude. We didn't think much of it. Around the same time, your doctor told us that you head was a little larger than a baby your age, but between your dad's ego and your aunt's large head, we didn't make much of it.

On Friday, September 12, just two days before you turned two months, your mom was changing you and discovered that your right thigh was extremely swollen. She immediately rushed you to the hospital at Saratoga where they x-rayed you. Unfortunately, they couldn't find the problem so they sent you to Albany. We spent that first night with the doctors trying to figure out why your right leg was causing you so much pain. They ran test after test, but couldn't get the answer--but they kept searching. A different doctor suggested you have a cat scan on you brain to make sure you didn't have too much fluid in it (which may be causing your head to grow too fast). Sure enough, she was right. You had fluid there, but unfortunately, when they did a different test (called an MRI) the next day, they found something else on your brain. They ordered more tests on Monday and found a similar mass on your right thigh that was causing all of your pain. We saw doctor after doctor on Monday and they told us news that we never thought we would hear about a two-month old--you had cancer. I have to keep saying it out loud and writing it down, because it's just too big to wrap my arms around if I keep it in my head. When we heard that news, it was like the floor had dropped out from beneath your mom and me. Life just stopped...

We spent that day mostly crying--it was the worst day of our lives. Unfortunately, they couldn't tell us much more than that without getting "snippets" of the tumors that were growing in your leg and thigh. We spent the rest of the day trying to deal with this news and whispering in your ear that you were going to be all right. By this time, you were spending nearly the entire day sleeping because the pressure in your head was getting so great. The good news was that they were going to perform surgery on Tuesday to help relieve some of that pressure and also to get those snippets that they needed to help find out what we were up against.

On surgery day, your mom and I were scared because we didn't know how you would handle surgery. We knew they were going to be putting you to sleep and then putting something in your head to help relieve that pressure and grab those snippets. That's not something anyone should have to go through, much less a two-month old. We chose to show our fears in two ways--your mom was sad for you and wanted you to be comfortable. Your dad was angry (he does that well) and wanted to fight whatever was inside your body. We were thrilled that after three hours of surgery, they were able to create another hole in your brain to let that fluid drain out and also safely grab those snippets from your head and leg. When you got back to your hospital room, your beautiful blue eyes were wide open and looked around for hours. How painful the first two months of life must have been for you that you didn't want to even keep your eyes open. Did the world look different to you? Did you really see your mom and dad for the first time? It was so nice to see our baby boy finally seem content. Yes Will, Tuesday was a happy day.

Be brave
Be strong
We love you...

WEDNESDAY, SEPTEMBER 17, 2008

Will,

I woke up this morning and headed to the hospital like I've done each morning for the past five days. I'll be honest, when I wake up each morning and think about where I'm about to go, I want to run the other way. I walk across the bridge to the hospital and I'm not even aware of what's around me. It's like the world is still going on, but I'm in this narrow path and can't hear or see anything else around me. As angry and then happy as I felt yesterday, I woke today and just didn't have it. Fortunately, your mom was the strong one today.

I took you today to a series of tests--you had your third MRI in four days, another cat scan, and something called a bone scan. As I was sitting in the waiting room, I discovered it's never a good idea to sit alone during these times. Your mind just races in a thousand different directions. Will, am I strong enough to fight with you? I know you are and I want to be there with you but I've never been so scared in my entire life. I just can't understand why this happening to such a sweet little boy and why your mom and I are being tested like this. I tell you every day to be ready to fight and then I sit in a waiting room with tears in my eyes and question my ability to take that walk across the bridge to the hospital every morning. I am so sad for you that it hurts in a way that I have never felt before. I know I have to fight with you and hope that strength will come to me when you need it the most.

Tomorrow is such a big day for all of us. I'm already writing it down in my calendar as the worst day of my life (replacing the recently recognized Monday). Your mom and I are preparing for the worst, praying for the best, and at peace with something in between. We don't know what Dr. Porter will tell us tomorrow, but all signs point to you being in a fight for your life. When you see doctors and nurses with tears in their eyes as they stop by to say hello or ask if we need anything, you know that the news is going to hit your mom and dad like a punch in the gut. The fight begins on Friday and we'll be right there next to you every step of the way. You are in the amazing hands of doctors and nurses that want nothing more than for you to be able to tell people some day that you are a cancer survivor.

Just know that you have your mom and dad, Ben and Max, grandparents, aunts, uncles, cousins and hundreds of other people all saying an extra prayer tonight for you.

Be brave
Be strong
We love you...

THURSDAY, SEPTEMBER 18, 2008

Brave Will,

I told you yesterday that today was going to be tough. We went into today prepared for the worst and sadly, that's what we got. You were given a raw deal, my baby boy and were forced to fight what appears to be a losing battle.

We were told this morning that while the diagnosis had not been completed, it appeared to be something bigger than we could have imagined. Your mom and I sat next to you in bed and just cried along side each other. I looked into your big eyes and you stared right back at me. You don't even know why the tears were there and that hurts but also comforts me at the same time. But you also don't know how difficult your challenge is and now we're forcing you to fight for something you know nothing about.

It appears as though you have a cancer known as rhabdoid. Your doctor indicated this is very rare and only 3% of all brain tumors are diagnosed as this type. Because it's so rare, they've had a difficult time finding a way to treat it. She told us that despite all the medicines we can try to give you, this kind of cancer usually figures out a way to fight through it and continue to grow. She told us that your time with us might be short. I just can't comprehend all of this. I can't figure out why every day we just keep hearing bad news. Why were you chosen for this fate? You come from such a loving family, why is this happening to us? What test are we being given?

Your mom and I talked today about how our life was on a path and now we're going on a different path in a different direction. This is what life has given us and we're at peace with that. We hope you can travel on that path for as long as you decide you can be there with us. No matter what, we're permanently on that path and will continue to try to discover why we're heading this way now.

Your mom and I decided tonight that we'll be sad for only a little while longer and then we're going to be strong. We know that everyone who loves, cares, and prays for you will need our strength. We also know that the fight for your life will also require every ounce of strength we have. As your doctor told us tonight, in a couple of weeks, you'll be able to tell us if it's a winnable fight and if it isn't, we're going to make all the right decisions to make sure we cherish every moment we have with you.

I thought that I would be writing this journal for you to read when you got older, and I'm beginning to realize that despite everything that you are doing to stay healthy, that goal may not be reachable. But I'm going to keep going because I need you to know that your mom, brothers, and I have not given up hope yet. This is your legacy Will and I want everyone to remember you. We've had doctors and nurses cry with us in our room today--they can't comprehend how something like this happens. Nevertheless, all of them have said that they will never forget you. I hope you realize that in your short life, you have had such an impact on so many people who didn't even know you existed seven days ago.

So what happens next? Tomorrow, Friday, we start our fight. You'll have surgery to insert a tube in your chest that will allow the doctors to give you medicine to see if we can beat this beast that's living inside of you. Once you are out of surgery, you'll begin chemotherapy for about five days. In about a week or so, we're praying that we'll see some sign of improvement. If we do, then we know there's a least some hope. We're still not sure when we'll bring you home. Your mom and I are very nervous about how your brothers will react to seeing you sick and we don't want to make them scared or nervous. At the same time, we long to be a family of five again and do things that a "normal" family will do. It's a decision we'll have to make when the time is right...

Your mom and I love you so much that we promise you that for however long you're with us, you will be comfortable and never suffer for a moment. You will tell us and we will take direction from you.

We can't change the last seven days and we can't make what's inside you go away. We can't take all of those poisons and put them in our bodies because god knows that's what we both want to do. All we can do is lie beside you, pray for you, be strong for you, and take each day as it comes.

Be brave
Be strong
We love you!

FRIDAY, SEPTEMBER 19, 2008

Brave Will,

My previous letters to you have allowed me to really reflect on what this past week has been like for your mom and dad. Only today, after reading the thoughts and well wishes from everyone who has read your story, did I realize just how much your story has touched so many people's lives. Your mom and I are so thankful that we have hundreds of people thinking about you and praying for you.

Today felt like a black cloud had been lifted away from us. For the first time in a week, the pain that had been inside of me slowly went away. Your mom and I talked last night and decided that we could either stay really sad or be strong--either way you would still have cancer. We know there will be moments to be sad at various times down this path, so there is no point in having sadness run our lives. So today, we felt strong and let others who visited be sad because they needed to be more than us. Here's the thing Will, your mom and I feel we've taken you as far as we can go. At this point, we stand beside you, support you, and give you strength, but we have turned you over to the capable hands of our doctors and nurses. We are all at the mercy of their wisdom. We made a difficult decision this morning--we could either accept the fate that you have been given or we could make an all-out effort to see if we could beat this thing. We know it won't be easy on you, and we struggled with our decision, but your mom and I thought that if there is still a miracle left in that tiny little of body of yours, we needed to give you every opportunity to share it with the world. I know there will be times over the next few weeks where we are going to wonder if what we decided was the best for you, and there are certainly no guarantees that what we decided is going to make your fate any different. We just know that if we don't give you that chance, that one shot, we will always wonder, what if?

So as I am typing this, I am watching them administer your first dose of chemotherapy. They are trying to tell us what they are doing to you, but it is all so overwhelming. Your Uncle Bill (or Ubil) gave us the best comparison for what is happening. He told us to picture the ocean where the waves slowly come ashore and wash away the debris leaving only the perfect shore. That's what we picture happening inside of you. You are going to be getting one thing or another for five straight days. After that is done, we wait and hope and pray. After about a week, you'll begin to tell us if the medicine is working. Your answer will guide us from there.

They told us today that you will be spending another month at the hospital until we can determine if your treatment is having an effect. We understand that this is the best place for you to get all of the care you will need to help you through whatever comes your way. Even though you have slept through most of today, you would be amazed at the number of people that have stopped in to wish you well, share their hugs and kisses, and just sit to support your mom and me. I simply cannot comprehend how many people your life has touched in such a short amount of time. You have inspired people to stop and think about their own lives and be thankful for the little things that we have all taken for granted for so long. We are truly blessed to be in the presence of such an awe-inspiring human being.

Be brave

Be strong

We love you!

SUNDAY, SEPTEMBER 21, 2008

(Letter from Mom)

Hello my sweet baby boy,

Daddy felt too exhausted to write last night, and while I don't have the gift to express myself like Daddy, I felt it was my turn to write to you. You had another surgery on Friday to put the port in your chest. I hate seeing it there, but I know it allows the doctors and nurses to help you without having to poke at your little body. I am trying hard to be strong buddy, but seeing what the Chemo is doing to your body is hard to watch. You and your Daddy are giving me more strength than you can imagine. Every time you open your eyes, I can't help but smile at you despite the way my heart is breaking.

I have always felt confident as a parent, and now I don't know what to do. I just want to hold you and feed you, yet those are the two things you want least. And while I know this isn't about me, I have never felt so helpless in my entire life. I knew you were a miracle from the day I found out you were in me. What a rough pregnancy, yet you made it through. You have been fighting since day one and although we are asking so much of you, we need you to keep fighting.

Your big brothers came to see you today. I could tell how nervous Ben was when he climbed up next to you. He asked Mommy and Daddy some tough questions. We wanted to protect him like we are trying to protect you, but we knew we needed to be honest with him. This is going to be a long journey buddy, but we are all on it with you.

Be Brave
Be Strong
We Love you!

SUNDAY, SEPTEMBER 21, 2008

Brave Will,

It's been a whirlwind of activity this weekend. There were so many friends and family of your mom and dad's that came to see you this weekend, that it never felt like we were alone (which is a good thing). They all came with a tear in their eye, but once they looked at you, saw how strong you looked and had a chance to talk to us, they all left with a smile on their face.

I got to spend most of today with your brothers. We went swimming in the pool, watched football and played with friends. I think things will get a little harder on your brothers now because they haven't had their mom and dad at home for over a week. We've tried to explain why to them, but it's been so much more difficult than we can bear.

We're going to try to do some things this week that feel "normal" to all of us. I'm certain this will only boost our spirits.

Today you received your second chemotherapy treatment. You reacted exactly as they would have wanted and we will continue to press forward. Tomorrow's treatment is going to pack a pretty big punch, and we're a little fearful of the effects, but we've seen you conquer so much already, I doubt you'll feel like tomorrow's medicine will feel like anything more than a mosquito bite. We've also started playing ocean sounds while you receive your chemo. It forces us to be reminded about the waves washing away the debris that Ubil told us about.

With all of the activity today, it felt good to take my mind off of everything that is happening in the hospital room. As I was sitting with all of these people, I thought about how it almost felt like you weren't as sick as you actually are. When I got back to the room and told your mom how I felt, I was disappointed because I know what the reality is. But as I told this to your mom, she said, "You know what that is? That's hope." She's absolutely right. Hope is not feeling as though the walls are closing in on us each and every day. Hope is getting small pieces of good news from the nurses throughout the day, insignificant towards your complete recovery, but still small battles that you will need to fight on a daily basis. Hope is watching you eat a 2 ounce bottle for the first time since Friday morning. Hope is having you look around the room while you are getting a bath. Those are the signs that show us that there is a lot of fight left in that little body of yours. We still are always conscious of the disease, but for today, my brave boy, today is a day for hope.

Be brave
Be strong
We love you!

MONDAY, SEPTEMBER 22, 2008

Brave Will,

Your mom and I finished the day together doing what we do every night. We sit next to you in the hospital bed and we read the powerful messages that people have been leaving on this website. You have no idea how much this helps us wake up the next morning and brace ourselves for another day. Whether it's a family member, a friend, or someone we have never met, we're well aware of how much of an impact you have had in your short life.

Today, you received your third treatment. Because the fluids have turned you into a little marshmallow, you're a little behind in your treatment plan. The doctors have decided to give you a day off tomorrow to let the fluid drain a little more out of your body. Then, on Wednesday, you'll get a heavy dose of something we can't pronounce. Yesterday, your mom and I decided not to try and remember all of these names and instead refer to them in kinder tones. Why refer to something with the name "toxin" in it? Instead, over the last three days you've gotten a treatment of "Yellow Flower" and "Ocean Water". On Wednesday, you'll get something we now call "Desert Sunset". Doesn't that sound better for you?

A couple of people commented to us today that your mom and I were in "a good place" right now. That's how we both feel. Our hearts ache every day but the sadness has lifted ever so slightly. We know sadness isn't going to cure your cancer, so we need to find another way to conquer this. Your mom and I are very aware of what could happen to you and we are prepared for anything at this point. But we also know that together, for the first time, we truly believe we have the strength to make the right decisions each and every day, no matter how difficult they may be. After a week of having things decided for us by forces we cannot defend you against, we are now able to decide things to help you in your battle.

Your mom was able to hold you in her arms up against her for the first time in over a week today. Your eyes were wide open looking around and you looked as content as the first day she held you on July 14th. I imagined you without pain and fear while she was doing this. It was an image I wasn't sure I would see again and it will be an image I will never forget.

Be brave
Be strong
We love you!

TUESDAY, SEPTEMBER 23, 2008

Brave Will,

I know that during this journey, there will be good days...and bad days. And then there will be something we'll call "even days", when the news is neither good nor bad. Today was definitely an even day. You got a day off from your treatment so that you could continue to let some of the fluids flow out of your body. It was so nice to see you look like a little baby boy again and not a shar-pei puppy. We decided last night to reduce the amount of morphine being given to you. We thought you would be able to handle it and that you would have a little more awake time. We were right on both--what good parents we are!! You had some great awake time tonight and spent nearly four hours looking around the room and at the faces of those visiting. You were even finally able to check out the faces of the nurses and doctors who had been poking and pushing you for the last few days. Your mom and I are pretty certain that you are taking mental notes of faces and names to act out your revenge when you're up and moving--there's a name for this type of list, but I know we've got some kids reading this, so we'll keep that between you and me.

"Even days" don't bring earth-shaking news, but then they also don't bring heart-breakers either. They're just days when we can enjoy you for who you are and not think about what's going on inside of you. Even days allow your mom and I to appreciate those that come to visit, even those we haven't seen in a while, but still carry a friendship that has never ceased. Even days allow us to focus on other things that up until last week seemed so important--the bills that need to get paid, the decisions on a house that still needs to get built, Ben's open house night, and how Max did at his pre-school today. These are distractions that we don't always allow ourselves to get distracted by when we're having one of those bad days I told you about.

But even days don't always match how your mom and dad are feeling. We each have something called a mood, and despite how good or even a day is, your mom and I don't always have the mood to match this. We've become quite good at knowing how to work together so that if one of us is having a tougher day and is in a bad mood, the other one uses his/her strength to lift both for the day. We know we need one of us to use the other, so we usually start the day by asking--"good or bad this morning?" If your mom is feeling a little down, then I know I'll need to be a little more positive. If your mom is feeling good, then I know I can let my mind drift a little to the sad side. We're still learning to find this delicate balance, but I suspect in no time we'll have it down to a science.

We're both off to sleep now. You've got a big day planned for tomorrow as you receive your "desert sunset". It's difficult to guess whether this will be a good, bad, or even day, but I do know it's an important day for your treatment and road to recovery. I think we'll both need to be in a positive mood and send you nothing but encouraging thoughts throughout the day.

Be brave
Be strong
We love you!

WEDNESDAY, SEPTEMBER 24, 2008

Brave Will,

Shhhh...I'm going to tell you a secret, little buddy, but I don't want you to get too excited...you had a pretty good day today and for the first time in over a week, the news that came out of our room was positive.

Your mom and I were getting ready to leave the hospital room together for the first time in over two weeks to go to your brother's kindergarten open house. Just as we were walking out, your doctor came in to examine you. Like all of us, she was impressed by how much the swelling had gone down in your body. But what she told us next really made us stop and listen. As she was examining the leg that has been infected with tumors which have kept you from moving it for two weeks, she noticed it had changed. The cancer is still there, but it was definitely not the same at it was four days ago. In a nutshell, the medicine that has been going in to your body is having an effect. How big of an effect, we won't know for a little while longer, but something is definitely happening. On top of all of that, this news came even before you got your "desert sunset" tonight. This is the medicine that is designed to go after the tumor that is located in your brain. So we're thinking, if those other medicines have been attacking your leg and the desert sunset attacks your brain, maybe we really do have a fight on our hands. When we came back later tonight and watched you move around in your bed and watched those muscles in your right leg working to move it ever so slightly, I know we're not far from seeing you eventually lift that that leg to show us what we've all known--you've only just begun to fight.

But here's the thing, and it's the reason why this is a secret, this thing is going to be a rollercoaster ride. Your mom and I loved the fact that we walked out of that room tonight with a smile on our face, but we're both grounded enough to know that this is merely a small hurdle. What we're all faced with is a marathon not a sprint. We'll gladly take these small victories, but in the end, we have our eyes on a much bigger prize and today, for the first time, we feel we might actually get there.

Here's the even better news. In just about a week, you have amassed an army of supporters that are fighting on your side. I was telling your mom today that just as the cancer has been spreading throughout your body, our army has been spreading too. It started with family, then spread to close friends. Over the past week, we've watched as its spread to long-lost friends, current and former colleagues, high school and college classmates, and people we've never met. Every day, we can tell when your story has reached a new faction of your army because of the messages that people have been leaving for you. So while the doctors have been giving you medicine to prevent your cancer from spreading, your army of supporters is still growing and I think we've got the cancer outnumbered.

So, with the last drop of desert sunset tonight, you've finished your first round of chemotherapy. You'll continue to get medicines for the next few days to help build your little body back up to where it needs to be, but the weapons you need to fight the disease are now part of you. I ask you, Brave Will, to allow those medicines to do what they need and while the next week may be painful for you, know that these medicines are going to do what they have to do to get you back home again.

When I left your room tonight, your eyes were open wide as your head lay upon the pillow and you looked so peaceful. Know that tonight, when my head eventually hits the pillow, I'll be at peace too...

Be Brave
Be strong
We love you!

THURSDAY, SEPTEMBER 25, 2008
(Letter from Mom)

Hello my sweet baby boy,

Your Daddy went to work today for the first time so it was just the two of us. I was scared to be alone with you at first. I wasn't sure if I had it in me to be strong enough on my own. You must have sensed it like your Daddy does, and you were strong enough for us both. You continued to move your "bad" leg, had tummy time, cooed, and let me hold you for hours. I can't believe I am saying this, but the best part of the day was changing your stinky diapers. For the first time in 13 days, I was able to lift both legs to change you. You didn't flinch like usual, and at that moment I felt like there were no tubes, no cancer, just a regular day with my baby.

I continue to be nervous with you and try to remember that you are not made of glass. We may be able to go home next week. While this news brings me joy, I am nervous at the same time. I want to find our "new normal" at home, but am unsure of how I can care for you the way the doctors and nurses have here. I also need to figure out how to be the best Mommy to your big brothers while pouring so much energy into you. They have many questions, sweetie, and I want to be sure that I can answer them honestly while not scaring them at the same time.

As I write this, Daddy is lying by your side holding your hand while you coo. A sound we never thought we'd hear. I always knew I picked a good husband, but baby boy, you have an incredible Daddy. I look forward to the day many years from now when you question just how much he loves you and I can show you these letters that he writes you.

You will continue to get fluids tomorrow to ensure that Dessert Sunset washes out of your body. I envision it pulling the cancer away from your sweet body. Ben asked me if it goes back into outer space when it disappears. I told him that I would ask the doctors. However, with how you have been amazing us each passing day, perhaps you can tell him yourself someday.

I love you so much sweetie, and am proud to be your mommy.

Be Brave
Be Strong
We love you!

THURSDAY, SEPTEMBER 25, 2008

Brave Will,

I don't want to steal your mom's thunder because I'm so glad she got a chance to write to you tonight. However, writing to you each night has become one of the most important parts of my life.

Today was the first day in over two weeks that I didn't spend with you from sun up to sunset. I decided to go back to work today. It was extremely hard to leave you and your mom, but I knew that you were in a safe place and that your mom would watch every breath you took today.

It was a little strange being back at work because for the last two weeks, my job has been to protect and stand beside you. It took me a while to feel like I belonged there again, but it was good to feel a little "normal" for just a little while. Your daddy is lucky to be working at a place where I am part of one enormous family who has been watching your progress every day. I feel fortunate that even when I can't be at your side, I get constant strength from those around me.

Tomorrow, I'll spend the day again by your side. Your mom and I are going to watch you very closely tomorrow and over the weekend to see if we think you, well...actually "we", are strong enough to bring you home next week. I have the same worries that your mom wrote about so we'll need to ask the doctors some important questions tomorrow. At this point, I have little doubt that whatever we decide will be the right decision for you.

Be brave

Be strong

We love you!

SATURDAY, SEPTEMBER 27, 2008

Brave Will,

It's a marathon and not a sprint. That's what your mom and I need to keep telling ourselves. After two really good days where we saw lots of positive signs, yesterday was a struggle for both of us. Neither one of us had the strength last night to write to you, so we figured we would both try to sleep and give it a shot this morning. Last night was the first night in over a week that we have both slept in the room with you because neither one of us wanted to leave you.

Yesterday, the doctors found that the levels of "desert sunset" that were left in your body from Wednesday were still higher than they would like. They continued to put fluids into your body to get the medicine out. Unfortunately, when they put all of that fluid in, it makes the swelling increase in your little body and puts pressure on your leg, which has made you as uncomfortable as you have been all week. We know it has to be done to get you back to where you were earlier this week, but it's been hard for your mom and I to see you cry so much when we try to move you or pick you up.

We feel like we've taken a step backward. It's exactly what the doctors prepared us for and told us what to expect, but it's still hard to see. Your mom and I really felt at our weakest last night and we know that's not what you need from us right now. We just keep hoping that we have turned the corner, yet we know that's a long way off. Days like yesterday are what our life is now and we have to be prepared better for them in the future. While we're tiring, weakening, and thinking about how long we can do this for, we know you haven't given up yet, so that's what keeps us going. Thank you for giving us the strength every day.

Be brave
Be strong
We love you!

SATURDAY, SEPTEMBER 27, 2008
(Letter from Mom)

Hello my sweet baby boy,

Daddy and I spent some time together last night to go to a concert. I could see the place from your hospital window, so that was the only way Daddy could get me to go. It was acoustic music so it left me with a bit too much time to think. I am trying so hard to take it day by day and not look beyond that. However, I let my mind drift last night and have been feeling very down ever since. Perhaps you are sensing that and therefore continued to have a bad day today. The doctors and nurses (and daddy) keep assuring me that it is what chemo does, but I just can't stand not being able to fix you up and comfort you. As I type this you are lying with me in just a diaper to try to bring your fever down. You are also not giving up your blood easily so you are continuing to get poked. I am praying you get a good night of sleep my sweetie. Your body needs time to rest and allow the desert sunset to leave your body and take away the cancer cells with it.

I am amazed at all the wonderful things people are doing for you and our family. The love and support continues to carry Daddy and me through these days. Daddy was telling me how, because of you, he and I will no longer see flaws in people (which we shouldn't have anyway), but we will only see their hearts. This has happened for us already, and we can't thank you enough for changing our ways. Many people have come to see you again today from near and far. The positive energy they bring is so incredible and exactly what we all need.

Your brothers are staying at the hotel tonight, so while daddy stayed with you, I had dinner with them and put Max to bed. It felt wonderful being with them, yet I couldn't walk fast enough to get back to you.

I am off to bed now. I feel so very lucky to get another night to snuggle next to you and whisper all my secrets in your ear. I love you so much sweetie and just want you to be comfortable.

Be Brave
Be Strong
We love you!

SUNDAY, SEPTEMBER 28, 2008

Brave Will,

It seems as though in this life you are living, you are just being thrown obstacle after obstacle. I'm having a hard time understanding how over the past two weeks you have been unable to catch even one break. It's so incredibly frustrating and I'm feeling totally helpless...

About an hour ago, we found out that the reason your fever reached 105 degrees last night was because you have a really bad infection. It just feels like a no-win situation. If we hadn't given you the chemotherapy, the cancer would have gotten the best of you. Now, because of the treatment we decided to give you, there's another enemy waiting.

Basically, it comes down to this. When you received your desert sunset on Wednesday, we knew it was going to pack a punch. It has dropped your normal blood levels way down and made your body susceptible to infection. With any chemo, there's always a risk for infection, and unfortunately, in this case, you were an unlucky one. What makes it even more complicated is that you need more white blood cells to fight this infection, but the medicine they need to give to increase your white blood cells cannot be given until you flush all of that desert sunset out of your body, and for some reason, your body doesn't want to seem to let go of it. Right now, they are putting different medicines in your body to try and fight off that infection and we're praying they can hold it off until your body can start to naturally take care of those nasty bacteria.

Your mom and I are simply devastated. On the one hand, if we hadn't tried to give you the type of treatment we did, you would have been fighting a losing battle. On the other hand, because of this course of treatment, we're afraid now we've put you in even greater harm. We know we did what was best for you, but was it too much for your body to take? Did we do things that may shorten your life as a result?

Tonight, we both sit in silence with our thoughts. We're not scared about what's going to happen to you in a year, a month, or even tomorrow. We're scared about what is happening to you minute by minute. We're going to muster up every ounce of strength we have left to get you through this next battle, and we'll be watching you every step of the way. I love you for always, my littlest one.

Be brave
Be strong
We love you!

MONDAY, SEPTEMBER 29, 2008

Brave Will,

It's just you and me tonight, kid...Your mom is back in the room getting a much, much needed night's rest. Last night, she told me that I need to get comfortable holding you. I had been avoiding this out of fear of hurting you, unsure that I would be able to give you the comfort you need.

But tonight I decided that I would lay on the bed with you and let you sleep soundly on me. It was everything I could have imagined. I'm glad you decided you wanted to watch the football game. I was afraid to ask you, but you brought it up and how could I tell you no??

It brought me back to last month when you would lay on my chest and just sleep so soundly, before any of this mess had entered our minds. Tonight, I didn't even think about the pain you were feeling. All I could hear was you snoring away in the deepest sleep, like you didn't have a single care. I'm not sure there is a more beautiful sound in the world than listening to an infant snoring and snorting as they deeply sleep. I could listen to it all night...

I'm glad your mom told me to do that. I really need to enjoy every minute, day, week, month, and year of my life with you. I promise not to be so scared to be around you and not to treat you as though you were made of glass. You're my little warrior who has handled pains greater than anything I could ever have imagined. I'm sure there is nothing in my arms that can take away the pain, but tonight, it sure felt like I could.

Be brave
Be strong
We love you!

TUESDAY, SEPTEMBER 30, 2008

Brave Will,

Your doctor spent some time with us today talking about the rollercoaster ride that has become your life. Today was a prefect example of how quickly things can change. Within an hour of being awake today, your room was filled with doctors and nurses. They were very concerned about your breathing, which had slowed way down. There was/is some concern that the tumor in your brain might be putting some pressure on your "command center" which affects your breathing and heart rate. They took lots of pictures of you today--cat scans, MRIs--to see if they could tell if the tumor in your head has grown. While they couldn't tell for sure, they are certain that your behavior has changed. Maybe it's the infection causing this, maybe it's the fluid that is increasing in your head again (that they did see), or maybe, and sadly, it's the tumor in your head that is not being affected by the chemotherapy.

We can only be observers at this point. We'll watch your breathing all day and night to see if anything changes. We'll watch your chest to make sure it is still moving up and down at a regular rate. We'll watch your beautiful big eyes to make sure they are staying focused on us. We'll watch...and then we'll wait. In a few days, we should be able to better determine what is causing you to act this way and then we'll know where to go from there.

Your doctor talked to us tonight about some pretty big decisions that we may need to make in the very near future. They are decisions that no mom and dad should ever have to think about, and I'm sure I'll tell you more about them when and if they are needed. But what she told us two weeks ago is no different than what she told us today. The biggest difference is that we get the feeling that we are closer to having to make those decisions, and Will, that is very frightening to your mom and me.

So tomorrow, we'll see where the rollercoaster is headed next. Will it go up? Will it go down? I don't know about you buddy, but I'd prefer to get off of this ride altogether.

Be brave
Be strong
We love you!

Brave Will,

If I've learned one thing about hospitals over the last three weeks, it's that there is a lot of waiting. That's what today was basically about. You continued to take your antibiotics to fight the infection, but you continue to be fever-free for a third day. You continued to take medicines to allow you to pass fluids through your body, including the infamous desert sunset, which I am proud to tell you, has finally made its grand exit from your body. But besides all of that, today we waited and we watched. You continued to give us some signs that things aren't quite right in your head, but right now, it's nearly impossible for the doctors to tell your mom and me what is causing it. You see, Will, you have a smorgasbord of things going on in your body right now. There are tumors, fluids, medicines, and infections all competing for our attention. We need to slowly take each one off of the table to really determine what is happening and just how serious things are. We're hoping that those little things you've been doing will stabilize over the next few days, and that your counts that were lowered by the chemotherapy will slowly climb back up. When this happens, we should be able to better sort things out with the doctors.

Your day saw the addition of a huge contingent to your army. The middle school students at Mechanicville, where your mom and dad once taught, made origami cranes that we can hang all around your room. A wonderful teacher that worked with us brought two huge boxes of these beautiful birds that her students had made in class. The name of the birds tells it all--Will's Winged Warriors. There are over

250 of these birds that we will have looking down on you in your room to guide you through your journey.

Your mom and I want to thank you for a couple of special things you did today that showed us that you're not ready to give up. They may not seem like a big thing to you, but you have no idea what impact it has on us. First, you let your mom give you a tubby. Now I know you didn't enjoy it nearly as much as your mom did, please know that by letting your mom and I do those "normal" things, you fill us with so much joy and hope that allows us to keep going from day to day.

Then, tonight, you did some even better things. First, while I was lying next to you in bed, you took your pacifier for the first time in days. Those little sucking sounds that you make with your pacifier tell us that your brain is still sending you signals which is what the doctors are looking for. Then, for your final act, you took a bottle for the first time in almost a week. Your mom was able to feed you nearly an ounce, which is very little for most two-month olds, but for your mom and dad, it felt like a grand feast. These are the things--giving you a bath, giving you a pacifier, feeding you a bottle--that your mom and I took for granted last month, but that we will now cherish for a lifetime. So thank you, little buddy, for making us feel like a mommy and daddy today. I can't wait to see what you have in store for us tomorrow...

Be brave
Be strong
We love you!

THURSDAY, OCTOBER 02, 2008

Brave Will,

My goodness, my little man, you sure do know how to fight. Just two days ago, I was afraid that you had been entered into a fight, yet you weren't being allowed to throw any punches. The doctors and nurses feared for your life. Today, just days later, you showed us just how unpredictable each day of your life is going to be.

While there is no question that there are some serious and critical problems in your head that will need to be addressed very soon, your mom and I and the countless visitors you had today, all saw someone different lying in that bed today. The swelling in your body that had been lingering for nearly two weeks was all but gone. Your appetite that had left you for the last week was back in a small way today as you set your weekly record for bottle consumption by chugging back nearly two ounces. What thrilled us the most today was how you were working ever so hard to lift that little right leg that has pained you for three weeks--you actually were able to raise is ever so slightly off of the bed. I could tell you wanted to move it as freely as you do its companion, and I have no doubt, that with your determination, you will be doing this in a matter of days.

You truly are a fighter, buddy. There is no question in my mind now. We know we've asked you to absorb so many big blows over the last few weeks, and I have no doubt that when you let us know you've had enough, your mom and I will grant you that wish.

The prognosis for your recovery hasn't changed, but I don't get the feeling you are ready to quit, so your mom and I are going to call on you again to continue to show us improvement. We won't be able to go after the nasty tumor and fluid in your head until we see you recover from all the chemotherapy that has been put into your body. So we'll wait with you for the next few days to see if you're able to do it. If you can, then we'll give you every opportunity to battle this thing. It may mean more surgery, more medicines, and more sickness. But if you're up for it, your mom and I will be right by your side. You're still the long shot in this race, Will, but I'm still willing to put my money on your side.

The doctor told us two weeks ago that you were going to tell us how to proceed by showing us a lot of little signs. No doubt, this week, there have been mixed signals coming from you. However, I still believe that you still have more of a story to tell and I can't wait to write all about it...

Be brave
Be strong
We love you!

FRIDAY, OCTOBER 03, 2008

Brave Will,

Today marks three weeks since we were admitted into the hospital. While I'm amazed that we've spent three weeks here, at the same time, it feels like we have been here a lot longer. So much has happened in 21 days, and I'm still stunned by how different our lives have become in such a short time. It's difficult to say when we'll be able to leave, and this place has become such a natural part of our lives. We still long for the day when all five of us can continue our lives together outside of C714.

You continued to be a "normal baby" today. We watched as you got more and more comfortable moving that leg. For the first time in three weeks, you actually straightened your leg out. You are definitely, what the doctors call, stable. In the world of this type of disease you have, we've learned that stable is good. It doesn't always have to be about improvement, as long as you are stable, that's a good sign. We'll continue to look for signs of stability, and hopefully, a little improvement over the weekend.

You know, buddy, for three weeks, I've been doing nothing but talking about you. Tonight, I want to tell you about two other people who are just as brave as you are--your brothers Ben and Max. They both came to the hospital tonight, and we hadn't seen or talked to them since Sunday. Apparently, they are both too busy to talk to their mom and dad. When they came tonight, and we got a chance to talk to them and ask them how things were going, your mom and I realized just how courageous they both are too. They are being faced with a different set of challenges than you face, but for two little guys, those challenges can be quite difficult. Every day, they don't know where they are going, how they are getting there, and what is going to happen next. They get dropped off at school, picked up at school, eat dinner, go to bed, and there could be someone different doing that every single time. Your mom and I are so impressed with how they have helped us get through these last three weeks. They care so much about you, little man, that they are willing to do whatever it takes to allow your mom and me to be here whenever you need us. That takes a different kind of bravery, and we don't always get a chance to tell them that. Your mom and I are so thankful that you have two brothers that are right there with us as we continue on this journey. One day, you'll see how lucky you are too...

Be brave
Be strong
We love you!

SATURDAY, OCTOBER 04, 2008

Brave Will,

Did you notice how quiet things were today? You spent most of the day with just your mom and me. The three of us even took a nap together on the bed. It was so nice to sleep beside you for a little while today--we all slept so peacefully. I can't wait for a day when the two of us can take a nap on the couch on some lazy Saturday afternoon.

We remain in a holding pattern today but do have some concerns that we are eager to address. We need you to eat a little more, big guy. You are willing to take a bottle, but you aren't interested in eating more than a 1/2 ounce or so a few times throughout the day. You are starting to look a little less pudgy. While your mom and I would welcome someone telling us that about ourselves, for you, keeping weight on is going to be important in your recovery. The doctors said they may have to give you a little nutritional supplement to help you stay healthy, but we want to wait a couple of days to make sure that infection that was in you has left for good.

I guess the hardest part has been watching your little head swell with fluid yet again. I remember seeing you when you got out of your first surgery and how wide open your eyes were when they relieved all of that pressure. To know that you are back to that place again with the pain in your head is tough for us to see. It's even harder to know they can do something to help you, but can't do anything until you are feeling better. The waiting, as someone once said, is definitely the hardest part.

So for today, there were some highlights and some concerns, which has become par for the course during this stretch. We'll wait as patiently as we possibly can and hope that you soon become ready to begin the next round of your battle. Whether it's this week or the next, we'll be ready whenever you are.

Be brave
Be strong
We love you!

SUNDAY, OCTOBER 05, 2008

Brave Will,

Thank you so much for bringing your bright eyes and wonderful smile today when the photographer came to the room to take pictures of you, your brothers, your mom and me. We were able to turn our hospital room into a photo shoot and you were more than happy to pose for the camera. I am thrilled that we were able to capture so many precious memories of all five of us together today. These photos are going to be so important to us as we move forward in the weeks to come.

So buddy, we're in a bit of trouble right now and I'm really not sure what to tell you. The doctors came in today and saw some things that are really concerning them regarding the fluid in your head. Unfortunately, as I have told you, they can't do anything to fix it because you are not well enough for surgery. The time we need for you to recover may not come quick enough and even with the surgery, there's still so many issues that you are facing. It just appears that at this time, no matter what the doctors try, and what your mom and I decide to do for you, trouble just seems to be lurking around every corner we turn. If we get through this current obstacle, we know that something else will be waiting for us. At what point will you tell us that enough is enough? And when you tell us, how will we handle it?

I've been told many times over the past month things like: there is a plan for everyone; everything happens for a reason; we only are given what we are strong enough to handle. You know what Will--that all means nothing to me at this point. I don't even want to think about all those things. You know what I want? I just want to run away with my three boys and your mom and just put all of this behind us, and yet I know this isn't possible. We just can't escape this and your mom and I are struggling with why this is still happening to us.

We continue to try to be positive and try to support you with all of our strength, but it is so hard to do when it seems like we're getting punched in the gut every single time. There is no measure in this world to quantify just how difficult this has been. Your mom and I knew this would take every ounce of strength we had, but honestly buddy, this is so much harder than I could have imagined, and yet I cannot even comprehend how hard this must be on you.

So tomorrow, we'll start another week, and we'll have our hopes raised and dashed at least another 30 times, and I suspect I'll be sitting here a week from now still pondering how we'll get through it, no further or closer to having my whole family back together again.

Be brave

Be strong

We love you!

MONDAY, OCTOBER 06, 2008

(Letter from Mom)

Hello my sweet baby boy,

I dreamt about you all night. One of the times when I awoke your foot was on my shoulder. You kept moving it and kicking me (was I snoring?). I couldn't stop looking at your sweet little foot. I remember the day you where born. Daddy was holding you and I could see your hands so I counted your fingers. Later when I held you I counted your toes. Everything was perfect with you. Little did we know this beast was inside you. Yet, even now with all the tubes, the gauze on your head, your port, I still look at you and see perfection. I feel so lucky that I was chosen to be your Mommy. While our time together may be short, you my sweet boy will always have a piece of my heart with you. I say you have a piece, yet I feel as if my entire heart is breaking but need to save some for Daddy and your brothers.

Oh, buddy, Mommy is so nervous about your surgery tomorrow. The doctor needs to go back into your head to relieve pressure. The concern is that your blood counts are not high enough for you to make it through surgery, yet doing nothing runs the risk of infection. So my sweetie, the doctors and Mommy & Daddy feel this is the lesser of two evils. I know you are strong and I pray you can make it through tomorrow.

I do know that this is just buying us some more time, and there will never be enough time with you. I know we are asking so much of you, but I need to ask you to keep going.

Be Brave
Be Strong
We love you!

MONDAY, OCTOBER 06, 2008

Brave Will,

So I went into work today to clear my mind a little. Your mom called me during the day to let me know that they decided to go ahead with surgery tomorrow. On my drive home from work, I started thinking about a TV show called Quantum Leap. About fifteen years ago, when I was in college, reruns of Quantum Leap would come on at 11:00 every morning. I don't know that I or any of the guys that I lived with were terribly enamored with the show, but for whatever reason, if you came home from class at 11:00, it was always on and we were too lazy to change the channel. At any rate, the show featured a guy named Sam who would go back in time and try to do things that would change the future. Throughout the show, his sidekick Al would appear with this little gizmo that would tell Sam how he was changing the future depending on actions he was taking. So why was I thinking about an obscure show from the late 80's? Well, after your mom told me you were having surgery tomorrow, I was wishing I had a guy like Al that could come in to our room and tell us what the percentages would be if we decided to have the surgery tomorrow versus waiting to see if things would get better on their own. Wouldn't life be easier that way? For days I've been telling you that you are not well enough for surgery, and then, in an instant, everything changed. The risks, they say, are simply too high to wait any longer for you to get better on your own. And while risks associated with surgery are incredibly high, not doing anything at all would certainly lead to problems you would not be able to endure.

So tomorrow, we once again turn you over to the capable hands of the surgeons. I do believe that we are doing what is best for you at this time and I hope that what we are doing isn't being selfish. But you see Will, in reality, your mom and I know we are being selfish. We want to be able enjoy you for as long as we can, whether it be days, weeks, months, or years. We promise we won't make you suffer and we'll do everything to make you comfortable, but we're asking you for a little more time. I continue to stare into your eyes every night when I lay next to you, and while I'm certain you are unaware of what is happening and just how critical your situation is, I also see that you have so much left to tell us in your story.

I don't know how much sleep your mom and I will get tonight and that's okay. It used to be a chore to have to get up with you in the middle of the night to feed or change you. Now, I would gladly lie beside you and listen to you take every breath and make every little sound until it was permanently etched in my memory.

We face a tremendous hurdle tomorrow, by far the biggest one yet. I know your army is going to be there beside you, as will your mom, dad, brothers, and family. I ask that you rest up tonight and gather every little bit of strength you have left and give us all you got. I know it's a lot to ask a two-month old, but I promise you that your mom and I wouldn't ask if we didn't think you could do it.

When we wheel you down to the operating room tomorrow, I'm going to whisper two words in your ear right after I tell you to be brave, to be strong, and that I love you. I'll say the words "Oh boy", which is what that Sam guy that I was telling you about earlier would say whenever he found himself in a new, unfamiliar situation. You're going to be in one of those situations tomorrow, but I hope as the surgery progresses, those percentages slowly start to sway in your favor.

Oh boy, indeed...

Be brave
Be strong
We love you!

TUESDAY, OCTOBER 07, 2008

Brave Will,

PHEW...

That sigh of relief you heard around 1:30 today was hundreds of people who have been following your every move. You again showed us just how amazing you are by ably moving through yet another brain surgery. The surgery that was performed on you is, relatively speaking, a fairly simple procedure. However, because of the amount of chemotherapy you received, your body was just not as prepared as the surgeons would like. However, they gently performed the procedure and were able to insert the shunt in your head to help you drain the fluid that has been building up. We were so relieved when we saw the doctor heading towards us in the waiting room with a smile on his face (no, I didn't hug him this time). You'll probably never be able to fully realize how difficult this day was for your mom and me. We had to do a lot of thinking last night and this morning--we wondered if you would have the strength to get through another surgery; we wondered if we would have you for another day; and we wondered if the reward outweighed the risk. Thank you for answering every one of our questions.

What makes the day so difficult still is that despite the stress and relief we felt today, we know that this was merely a sidestep and not a step forward. The surgery done today really doesn't get us any closer to beating the disease inside of you. In addition, there are still a lot of risks out there that we need to contend with. You are still very susceptible to infection as a result of the surgery and the doctors will need to watch you every minute. Basically, we know we still have a lot of work to do. But you know what today did? It gave us another day with you, and that is all we can ask for each and every day...just one more day. We'll keep making the decisions to help the doctors make this happen and as long as you're up for it, we are too.

So what happens next, Will? Well, we'll need some input from you to help us. We'll watch you over the next few days to make sure your body fights off any infections that may arise from the surgery today. Then we'll watch your blood counts to make sure they are rising to normal levels. At the same time, we'll look to see if your leg keeps improving and that you do all of the normal things that babies your age do--eat regularly, follow us with your eyes, and be as alert as you have been for the past week. If all of that happens, then you have told us that you are ready for the ocean waves again.

You aunt wrote last night that we would much rather be living in obscurity where no one know who you are. Your mom and I agree with her completely. But that is no longer possible--you are a rock star, folk hero, and role model for many, many people. Since this is where we are at now, we are just so thrilled that you have inspired so many people and are supported by hundreds, if not thousands, of people around the world. Your mom and I cannot thank them all enough, including the only people as brave as you are: the doctors and nurses at your hospital, the only people in this world that we would want to be your wingmen in this treacherous journey.

We bought ourselves some more time with you today. How much time, we won't know. All I know is that with every passing day, I am in awe of your courage and strength, and I can't thank you enough for being my Brave Will.

Be brave

Be strong

We love you!

WEDNESDAY, OCTOBER 08, 2008

Brave Will,

Tonight I want to tell you about something that your mom and I like to call our "new normal". You see Will, up until September 12th, we were living a fairly normal life. In the matter of days, our lives were shaken to the core and it's taken us quite a while to feel normal again. In fact, I don't even think there is such a thing as "normal" anymore. The normal that we were all accustomed to no longer exists. It's been replaced by what your mom and I refer to as the "new normal".

So today, we started to think about examples of the new normal. New normal is:

- o Being ecstatic when you take a 2 ounce bottle when just a month ago you were taking 4 and a half ounces
- o Asking the nurses what your counts are every morning, and being excited about your progress (even though we might not always know what it means)

o Getting to know doctors and nurses on a personal and professional level and willing to put all of our trust in their capable hands. This sometimes means letting you go from our arms.

o Being excited when the doctors tell us that you can move from the PICU back to the oncology wing, which is starting to feel like home to us, and at the same time, puts us one step closer to home

o Getting to know words like NPO, CBC, Hickman, CSF, MTX, shunt, colace and actually knowing what they mean and how they are helping you

o Walking into the hospital room in the morning, looking at your mom's eyes and knowing if today is going to be a good or bad day

These are the realities of our life now, our new normal, and we are ready to accept them into our routine. We know now that we'll need to be pleased with the little steps that indicate progress in your life. Our milestones will need to be set daily, not monthly or annually. We'll gladly accept every day that we get to stand by your side and help you in any way that we can.

Today, we again saw just how important your life is to people that aren't named mommy and daddy. We saw the joy in your nurses' faces when you made your triumphant return to the oncology wing, when just a day earlier, those nurses saw the worrisome look in our faces and wondered if they might ever see us again. We heard about the outpouring of love and generosity that hundreds heaped upon you at a fundraiser that was held tonight. Those people were all there because of your story and your spirit.

How does a two-month-old inspire so much joy and goodness in so many people? I'm not sure what your secret is but I sure am glad that I am lucky enough to be around you each and every day. There is something special about you, Will, and I'm fortunate enough to have a front row seat.

Be brave
Be strong
We love you!

THURSDAY, OCTOBER 09, 2008

Brave Will,

It's a little later then I normally write to you but after going to work today, I wanted to make sure I got to spend a little time with you tonight. Your mom and I will need to get used to this new routine and I know she'll get to spend a lot more time by your side than I will. But to be honest, if you had to choose between the two us, I would choose your mom too if I were you. There's really no one in this entire world like your mom. She would absolutely, without hesitation, give up everything in the world for you and your brothers. Being a mom is her true calling and I doubt there are many out there than can do a better job at it than her. She truly lives for her children and I am in envy of just how much love she can pour out each and every day for you, Ben, and Max. Just as we feel lucky to have you in our lives, Will, you should feel pretty lucky too to have a mom like her to stand beside you every moment of your life. I really don't know what we would do without her...

So while I was at work today, your mom was again by your side. She had the biggest smile on her face when I walked in the room tonight. She told me all about your day--how you had been waking up to eat just like normal, how people had brought some incredible pictures from your photo shoot to the room, and how you had spent the day looking and acting like a little baby boy. In fact, one of the nurses came in to the room because she didn't know who was crying--she hadn't heard you cry at all for over two weeks. The doctors even lowered your pain medicine because you are feeling a little better and they think you'll be able to function better without all the pain killers in your body. They are going to watch you for a couple of more days and expect to start your next round of treatment next week--the ocean waves will return.

We are so happy that you have done so well the past couple of days, but we're being careful this time. A few weeks ago, we watched you have a couple of good days and before the good feelings had a chance to settle in, we were dropped by bad news. This time, we're not thinking about anything more than how good of a day you had today. Tomorrow we'll do the same, and the next day, and the day after that. So while we know today was good, and we hope tomorrow is better, we also know that we have to expect anything and history has shown us that there are always going to be good days followed by some not-so-good days. But I'll be honest Will, I'm really liking these good days and hope that they'll last for a while...

Be brave
Be strong
We love you!

SUNDAY, OCTOBER 12, 2008

Brave Will,

I'm sorry that it's been a couple of days since I last wrote to you. The good news is that you have been doing pretty well and fortunately, have been steadily improving each day. The doctors are watching all of your counts and are preparing for your next round of treatment which could begin early next week. While we're not exactly sure if the first round of treatment had any effect on the tumors, we do know that things haven't gotten worse, which is your way of telling us that we should definitely give this another shot.

I didn't get to see you much at all on Saturday. I was able to go Other Ben and Darcy's wedding. I was so happy to be able to be a part of their special day especially after they have been by our side, supporting us, every single day over the past month. Your mom decided to stay with you while I went to the wedding. I can't blame her at all--it's really hard to be away from you for a long period of time. You tend to find yourself at the other place in body, but your mind is constantly drifting back to hospital, wondering what is going on. Eventually, you start to get antsy and all you can think about is getting back to see you. In a weird way, it's almost easier to be at the hospital with you than to be somewhere else. While I was able to see all of my closest friends and was able to celebrate such a special occasion, that drive back to the hospital was brutal. Whether I am at work, at a wedding, or just going across the street to eat, whenever I leave that place and start my trek back to the hospital, that reality kicks in and I think I might actually be sadder than if I had never left at all. I know I can't stop my life completely and I need these times to get my mind of off everything that is happening, but it's merely a temporary escape. I wonder when this changes, when your mom and I finally get to a point when we can do things as a family and not feel so nervous, anxious, scared, or sad. I'm sure it will happen eventually, but it can't come soon enough for me, and I suspect your mom as well.

So today, I think I'll just sit beside you and spend the day close by. It's just easier that way...

Be brave
Be strong
We love you!

SUNDAY, OCTOBER 12, 2008

Brave Will,

You are a tricky one to figure out, little man. Your mom and I spent most of last night and today trying to figure out just what is causing you to be so fussy. You appear to be uncomfortable, so we again raised your level of painkillers. However, when we do that, you don't eat as much and you are, what we like to call, "loopy". But if we drop your level, you appear to be in pain. It's tough because you're such a little guy. We don't know if it's pain from surgery, pain from the disease, or if you're just being cranky because you're a little baby. Since we don't expect you to be able to tell us, we are really guessing.

So today, we raised your morphine level to the highest it's been in a little while. We'll try to drop it down a little tomorrow, and a little more the next day as you get ready for the ocean waves again.

Your mom is going to sleep in the hotel tonight and get a much needed night's sleep. I'm looking forward to hanging with you in the room--we've got a choice of a baseball game and a football game. We're two lucky guys!

One of the doctors today remarked on how well your mom and I are handling everything. I wonder if we're either doing a really good job of fooling everyone or if we're really getting stronger. I tend to think that your mom and I are too much of a realist. We get how bad things are and therefore, when we talk to the doctors, we're really able to ask those tough questions that I bet a lot of moms and dads here are afraid to ask. It's probably helped your mom and me to be this way--to keep our guard up. We'll take the small victories as they come, but leave the thoughts of bigger miracles to others. We know you're still a long shot, but the doctor told us today that things can and do happen that are often difficult to explain. It's that way of thinking that makes our decision to start a second round of treatment this week pretty easy. We'll need you to get lots of rest over the next day or so and gather all of your strength and we'll all be ready to take another shot at the beast within...

Be brave
Be strong
We love you!

MONDAY, OCTOBER 13, 2008

Brave Will,

Thank you for taking care of me last night. I appreciate you reminding me that you were there throughout the night by sending out little grunts, cries, and sighs. When you knew I had been away for too long, you carried on so that I remembered to crawl in bed with you for a little while. Your mom and I are proportioned a little differently, so it was harder for me to crawl up beside you, but thanks for giving me just enough room so I could sleep next to you and lay my head right beside yours for a couple of hours this morning.

Your mom and I didn't spend too much time in the room today, for once. We chose to spend the day with your brothers and it was a great choice to make. We left you in the capable hands of your grandma and papa and knew that you were feeling just fine when we headed out the door. We got to take your brothers out to lunch and catch up on their lives a little bit. We miss them so much and it was great to spend time cutting their hot dogs, wiping their faces, and sharing their ice cream. After lunch, we put your brother Max in for a nap and took Ben over to our new house that is being built. He used a digital camera he just bought to take lots of pictures of the house. He can't wait to show you pictures of your room. We still have a long way to go before it is ready, but we can't wait to bring you home to our house. We know you'll find it as safe and cozy as we all think it will be. Your mom and I have had very little time to focus on the house. It's strange, all we could talk about before last month was the house. Then, for weeks after you got sick, we barely gave it a few minutes of thought. Now, we appreciate the diversion of it. We don't have the same excitement that we had before, but it's been a nice distraction and all we can do is think about how awesome it will be to bring you there when it is all done. We even put one of your Brave Will stickers in the rafters above your room so you would know exactly where to go when we finally get there. How our thoughts have changed--before, we were planning where to put the television and the dishwasher. Today, we looked for a place to put the Purell dispenser and air purifier. These are the modifications we would gladly make if it helps make you more comfortable at the new home.

While we were gone, the doctor came in to tell your grandma and papa that your next round of treatment would begin on Wednesday. There giving you an extra day because there is one more number that they test you for that they would like to see climb a little higher. They also want to give you more days to get a little more food in your belly. You've lost a little more weight than they would like, so they really want to see you eat more. So do me a favor tonight and tomorrow, don't be so self-conscious about your weight. If you want to pig out, then go for it, little man. We'll keep giving you the bottles if you keep chugging them down. I know formula isn't the best tasting stuff around, but there are some important goodies in there that will help your body grow and stay healthy.

I'm really eager to get the next round of ocean waves going. I'm crossing my fingers, as is everyone who now knows the name Brave Will, that this next round will have a positive effect on the disease in your body. The positive thoughts that may have escaped room C714 over the past few weeks will start to return on Wednesday and we'll use all of that positive energy to support you as the bell on the second round sounds...

Be brave
Be strong
We love you!

TUESDAY, OCTOBER 14, 2008

Brave Will,

It's getting late tonight, but I was unable to put you down all night. After I got home from work, I held you for a while and got to feed you twice. Your mom told me that you were eating well today but had some problems keeping the food inside of you. However, when I fed you tonight, you did pretty well the first time. Then the second time I fed you, not only did you finish an entire bottle for the first time in a long time, you also even started a second bottle. I cut you off because I was afraid of overfeeding you, but as I asked last night, you totally pigged out while I was with you tonight. Good job buddy! I have one simple explanation for this--you just needed your dad there to feed you. I know your mom likes to think that she's the one that you respond best to, but I think we showed her tonight. After we ate, we chilled out to a little Ray (I bought you his new CD today for your three month birthday) and you slept so peacefully on me. Despite the fact that I only got to see you for a few hours, it really felt as though I was with you all day.

I understand you had lots of people visiting you today, including a friend of your grandma and papa's that has known your daddy since he was born. Can you believe he drove all the way from North Carolina just so he could see you in person? I'm telling you, little buddy, you have this magnetic attraction. People just want to be around you, see how you look, say hello to you, and maybe even learn from you. It's pretty incredible for your mom and I to see day in and day out. You really are affecting people's lives in such a positive way and I'm so proud of you.

The doctors told us that one of your numbers was a little low, so they may wait until tomorrow afternoon or maybe even Thursday to start the next round of treatment. No worries though--we know you're ready to take the next step. In fact, I watched your "bad" leg move so much tonight; it really looked like you literally wanted to take the next step. It's clear you're on board now, ready to pull your beach chair right up to the coastline and let the ocean waves roll across your body...

Be brave
Be strong
We love you!

WEDNESDAY, OCTOBER 15, 2008

Brave Will,

Well, well, well...that was some surprise your mom and you had planned for me when I got home from work today. As I opened the door to leave the hotel and head over to see you, I couldn't believe my eyes. There standing in front of me at the hotel was you! My first thought was, uh-oh, did your mom bust you out of the hospital?!? But then she explained to me that your counts were high enough that you could leave the room for an hour. This was your first and last chance before the chemotherapy begins again tomorrow morning. Your mom and I didn't even know what to do--it had been over a month since we last were able to be out of a hospital with you. We took you outside to get a breath of fresh air in your lungs--did you feel how incredible an autumn night feels? The air is so crisp this time of year and I'm sure that clean air felt wonderful as it glided through your body. The fall has always been our favorite time of year, so we were happy that you got to experience it too.

I just know there will come a day soon when you will be able to spend even more time outside on your road to recovery, but for now, we've got some bigger mountains to climb inside that hospital. You're still on schedule to begin your treatment tomorrow morning--I think you start with "yellow flowers" again. The doctor has given all of the nurses the game plan and we're confident everyone is going to do their part to make sure everything goes as well as could be expected. It's quite a bit easier this time around for your mom and me (can't believe I called your treatment "easy"--you'd probably disagree with me). It's just that this time, we know what you're exposed to. We're expecting, but not hoping for, the swelling, the possible sickness, the risk of infection. You got the whole menu last time, so nothing should surprise us this time around. The doctors are going to try to figure out a way to reduce the amount of fluids so that you don't become a little puffball again, but also that there are enough fluids to flush the different medicines out of you. It's a delicate balance to strike and I hope we can keep you as comfortable as possible.

The next four days should, knock on wood, be relatively event-free. It's the aftermath that we have to watch closely. Nevertheless, we'll just sit and enjoy time with you while those ocean waves come crashing in...

Be brave
Be strong
We love you!

THURSDAY, OCTOBER 16, 2008

Brave Will,

The ocean waves have started to roll in and so far, so good, little buddy. You received your ocean water and yellow flower to start the second round of treatment today. Your mom played soothing ocean sounds while the yellow flower was given to you over a six hour period. It's a lot of fluids for your little body to take but so far you seem to be handling things a lot better than last time. You're not nearly as swollen and you even maintained your appetite throughout the day. There's really nothing more your mom and I could have asked for on the first day of treatment.

Tomorrow, you'll get your third medicine out of the four in this round. We haven't come up with a new name for it yet--maybe those watching your story will have some ideas. Then, after tomorrow, we get ready for the heavy hitter, desert sunset. If all goes well, you'll be done with this round by Saturday night.

I wish you knew how happy your mom and I are to see you responding so well. Can you tell by the look in our eyes, the mood in the room, or the calm and peace in our voices just how much you affect us every day? Our lives revolve around one simple thing--to make sure you are comfortable and peaceful each and every day. When you achieve that feat, you bring us absolute joy like you could never imagine. So even though you may not be able to express this to us, that sly little grin you show us every so often (though not often enough) tells us that you might just realize how incredible you make us feel every single day.

Be brave
Be strong
We love you!

FRIDAY, OCTOBER 17, 2008

Brave Will,

Well done, my little friend, well done. You successfully navigated through another day of your treatment. While there is a little bit of swelling, it's nowhere near the amount that you had last month in your first round. You have continued to do a good job eating and are passing the fluids out as quickly as your body allows (even on your mom sometimes). Today, you got two more medicines, names we can't remember or pronounce but that we will now call Autumn Harvest (because the harvest fills you up but the season passes quickly) and another name that was passed along by one of your supporters, Yvonne. The second one is called Hai Chao and is Chinese for "Ocean Wave". It's pronounced "Hi" and "Ciao", which also means hello (English) and goodbye (Italian). So we like to think of that second medicine as entering your body and then just as quickly leaving carrying the disease with it. They're both cool names, don't you think? Tomorrow, you'll get the same medicines, before finishing up with the Desert Sunset on Sunday.

Now here's the cool/scary part...Your doctor came in tonight and talked to us about the future. It's really the first time we talked about anything beyond a few days. We started talking about next week and whether we will be able to go home. We talked about the next round of treatment and even what we might do after that round. What this means to your mom and I is that the story we asked you to tell us during the first round of treatment has been a very positive tale. Your doctor is not the type to give us false hope at all, so the fact that she is contemplating future treatment plans, indicates that she has seen some good things over the past few weeks. By no means has your prognosis changed and we're not fooling ourselves into thinking it has. But at the very least, there are some signs that the treatments are having some affect on your disease, enough that there is no way we would consider not taking the next steps. But admittedly, we're all kind of entering some unchartered waters with these next steps. By this point we would have already known if the treatment they were giving you wasn't working, so the long shot is still alive in the race. We'll be working hard with your doctors over the coming weeks to make sure we make the right decisions to ensure you continue to stay healthy and comfortable. But really, for the first time, there might just be the smallest flicker of light at the end of that very long tunnel. It's still going to take a long while to get there and we may never make it, but we're going to sure as heck give it everything we have...

Be brave
Be strong
We love you!

SUNDAY, OCTOBER 19, 2008

Brave Will,

Great job buddy!

Overall, you had an awesome weekend. The difference in your reaction to treatment this time versus the first round is incredible. The amount of swelling has been minimal and you're doing an awesome job of getting rid of all of those medicines in your body. You received two days of Autumn Harvest and HaiCiao, and then today, you got the infamous Desert Sunset. We'll let that one sit inside you for a little while to let it do its job and then tomorrow, they'll give you some more medicine to get that out of you. If you remember, last month, you were a little reluctant to get rid of the desert sunset and that made the doctors a little concerned. So, we're hoping, with the swelling not being as bad, you'll push that out of you a little faster.

We're also thrilled that we were finally able to stop giving you morphine. You've been on that painkiller since we got here five weeks ago. However, it seems like the pain in your leg has gone down, so there was really no reason to keep you on the morphine. Now, the doctors warned us that there might be side effects, like being fussy and irritable. These also describe the typical habits of a 3-month old, so we'll have to figure out which is which. As long as you don't start swearing at us, start throwing things, or try to bum smokes from the nurses, I figure you should be able to kick the habit pretty easily. Dropping the morphine is another important step towards becoming a "normal" little baby (or at least a normal little baby who happens to have cancer). These types of things, as well as some other important developmental milestones (following us with your eyes, eating more, lifting up your head) will help tell us that you are ready to progress even further and maybe even go home for a little while. Your mom and I are admittedly a little scared to bring you home, but if the time is right and we know you are safe, then we realize this is something we will have to do so that all five of us can be a family again. But I'll be honest, I'm having a difficult time imagining life with you outside the safety net of the hospital. We've gotten so used to the nurses and doctors being there at a moment's notice, we're not quite sure what would happen if we were able to take you out of there. However, it's a decision we'll have to make, hopefully very soon, and I am confident, like before, that your mom and I will make the right choice.

Fortunately, we've got a couple of days before we have to think about that. We'll need to see you get rid of all of that desert sunset, continue to eat more and more, and fight off any impending infections. If you're able to do that, then your mom and I have got some thinking to do...

Be brave
Be strong
We love you!

MONDAY, OCTOBER 20, 2008

Brave Will,

Sleep well tonight little guy...You spent most of today awake struggling to get comfortable. We're assuming, since you can't tell us, that it's probably from a little bit of withdrawal from the morphine. When I got home tonight, your mom said that you had spent nearly the entire day awake. So I was glad to see you sleeping when I arrived.

You've pretty much already passed the desert sunset out of your body. What took nearly a week to do last month was accomplished in a little over a day this time. So that's the first hurdle to clear this week. Next, we need to see you eat more. A nutritionist came to see you today to talk to your mom about some strategies we could use to try and fatten you up. The doctors aren't going to let us take you home until they are certain you are taken enough nutrition in every day. So again, I encourage you to pig out. I understand that this is going to be even harder than before because the chemotherapy is going to make your belly feel very sick. Outside of getting you to eat some more, there isn't much else that is going to be asked of you this week, so you can finally relax for the first time in a long, long time. We'll keep a close eye on your temperature as your counts start to plummet, but beyond that, we just ask that you eat and sleep. So start tonight with a good night's sleep and we'll see you tomorrow, ready to tackle another day...

Be brave
Be strong
We love you!

TUESDAY, OCTOBER 21, 2008

Brave Will,

I guess at this point, nothing should surprise me anymore. We've hit the lowest of lows over the past few weeks and have had lots of peaks and valleys on this journey. That being said, today definitely made me stop for a minute. You see, Will, today was one of those good news/bad news days, and I'm trying to figure out if the bad news is really all that bad.

The day started with a visit from your doctor. She decided this morning that we need to make you stronger and waiting to see if you would eat more (especially now that the chemo was starting to kick in) was just not a good option. So they started you this afternoon on something called TPN (total parenteral nutrition). Basically, they're going to use that tube in your chest to provide you with more nutrition and calories than you have been getting through your bottles. In addition, they can use the TPN to give you lots of other things that you may be lacking like potassium and magnesium. So while we would love it if you would continue to feed from your bottle, we know this is the best thing for you right now. Also, you've developed a pretty nasty diaper rash that probably extends all the way inside your little tush. This is causing you a lot of pain, so they gave you some medicine to help with that and also some antibiotics to make sure that rash doesn't lead to an infection in your belly like last month.

So basically it all boils down to this--you're such a little guy and you have all of these little things going on inside of you that makes treating you each day a challenge for your doctors. There's so many things they are watching inside of you that they need to be around you nearly every second of every day. As a result, they want you to stay right where you are. So we won't be going home anytime soon. In fact, it looks like you'll be in the hospital for at least another two months. So I guess that's the bad news part. The good news is that they want to keep you so close because they need to make you stronger so they can keep fighting this disease with you. Really, for the first time, there's a long-term plan for you. We've heard a lot over the past few days about just how bad things got last month, to the point where no one expected there to even be a need for a second round of treatment. Whereas before, they were treating you day by day, now they are looking at a two-month plan for you. That plan includes letting you build your body back up after that last round of chemo and then, in about three weeks, giving you another round of high-dose medicine. If all goes well after that and you are still showing that you have that fight in you that we've all come to expect, then it looks like they may let the surgeons have another look inside your brain to see if they can take out some of that nasty tumor. It's a step that your mom and I know you have to take in order to get better, no matter how fearful we are of letting someone do this to you.

So I'm not sure how to feel tonight. On one hand, I'm absolutely thrilled that we're looking further down the road than we ever have. I'm thrilled that there is a plan and there is confidence that you will be able to get to those next steps. On the other hand, I'm really at a loss for how to pull things together on this new path we are on. Tonight I write to you from the hotel room with your brother Ben sleeping in the bed next to me and your brother Max sleeping in the crib on the other side of me. We know now that we have to be able to include them more in the next two months. We are certain of what our life will be over the next 60 days, and we need to make sure they are more of a part of it. Your mom and I are going to try and figure out a way to start a new temporary life down here in Albany that includes all five of us. It's not going to be easy, but we simply can't continue down this road without your brothers with us. They need us, just like you do. But more importantly, we need them. It hit me hardest tonight when I said out loud that two months from today was December 21st. Two months didn't seem that long until I realized that this would mean Halloween, Thanksgiving, and the Christmas season would all be spent in a hospital or hotel room in Albany. I know this is the absolute right thing to do for you, but it's hard to imagine how things will pull together during these next few weeks. I'm sure once we sort things out and establish a new routine, it will become a "new normal" just like before.

So while I'm sorting out what the good news was today and what the bad news was, I think I'll stop trying to over think things and just be happy that there continues to be news to report to you at all because that means that there are doctors still looking for ways to help you, there are people still out there praying and thinking about you, and there is a little brave soul name Will still fighting each and every moment...

Be brave
Be strong
We love you!

WEDNESDAY, OCTOBER 22, 2008

Brave Will,

So many things are going through my head right now that I'm not really sure how to get this all down on paper. Today was a memorable day, an amazing day, a day that left us completely stunned and it started with two words I'll never forget--"substantial reduction". What does that mean? Let me tell you...

While I was at work today, your mom called to tell me that when the doctors came in this morning, they were concerned because your heart was beating very fast. They were afraid that the shunt in your head was having difficulty, so they immediately order a cat scan STAT! (Your mom and I have grown fond of adding stat to the end of anything we want done). The CAT scan was done to see what might be going on in your head. When the doctors came in to tell your mom what they found, they told her that there was nothing to be alarmed about. But what they told her next has undoubtedly changed our entire perspective of this battle. The same cat scan found that not only were there no issues with your shunt, but there was "substantial reduction" in the tumor in your brain. I wonder if you got to hear the elation and joy in the room when they said that. Your mom and auntie cried, the doctors cried, and I bet there was lots of hugging. When your mom called me at work to tell me, my first words were "What?" and then just silence as my eyes filled with tears and I was unable to say any words. Buddy, this news is far greater than anything we could have expected or hoped for at this point in your treatment. True story--the person who did the CAT scan called your doctor to ask how long ago you had brain surgery to have some of the tumor removed. That person saw so little of the tumor left that he assumed you already had surgery to have some of it taken out!

After I heard that news, I could have climbed a mountain or run a marathon. For the last six weeks, we have asked you every day to tell us how things were going--to tell us your story. The sign you gave us today is like nothing I could ever have imagined. Your mom and I have this renewed energy that we didn't think we had left in us. If you need us to spend two months in the hospital with you, then that's what we'll do, without hesitation, without reservation and with total dedication.

It's hard to think about what's next with the way we felt today, but we know we have to keep thinking about those steps. We know we still have some post-chemo issues that have to be addressed. Now that we know how your body is responding to treatment, we want to be sure that no stone is left unturned in your recovery from the last round of treatment. That means watching for every sign of infection, shooing away those that might have the sniffles, trying to supplement your nutrition with whatever the doctors think will make you bigger and stronger. We're going after this thing, buddy, with a ferocious energy, and you know what, we're winning right now--Willem 1, Cancer 0.

Lost in the excitement of this incredible news was your television premier. A local news channel featured a story on you and told all about how incredible and inspirational you are. They talked about your brothers, your mom and I, and the thousands of people whose lives you have been touching on a daily basis. There's no doubt about it, people want to know all about you, Will.

I get ready to sleep tonight carrying as much hope as I have had for the past six weeks. You have surprised us with the brightest news we could have hoped for at this point. We know we still have a lot of work to do, but it's clearer than ever before that you are up to the challenge. In our eyes, regardless of what happens from here, you are our little miracle.

Thanks for the good news, my littlest son, we needed that...

Be brave
Be strong
We love you!

THURSDAY, OCTOBER 23, 2008

Brave Will,

Gosh it felt so good to have a smile on my face all day long. I'm simply walking on air right now and nowhere near ready to come down. You have given your mom and me the greatest gift we could have asked for six weeks into this thing. There are a lot of people walking around the hospital shaking their heads in disbelief with smiles on their faces. You've got 'em baffled buddy, and that's a very good thing.

So today, your mom and I did some "old normal" things. I went to work today and was the recipient of lots of high fives and hugs from many of the people in your army. Your mom left the hospital for a little while and volunteered in Ben's classroom today. Your brother felt pretty special having all that alone time with your mom. He was bouncing off the walls when I saw him this afternoon--it was clear he needed that "mommy time".

Things have definitely settled down with some of the issues they were seeing yesterday and we're grateful for that. I'm certain that as close as the doctors and nurses were watching you before, with the news we got yesterday, they're keeping an even closer eye on you now. There's no way they want any complications from the chemotherapy, knowing that we've got a fighting chance now.

I thought a lot about the "what happens next" question. Here's what I know about the cancer you have--it's not going to like what's happening to it and it's going to fight back. That's just what this type of cancer does. It's going to keep trying to grow, and your mom and I are prepared to hear that at some point. That being said, the impact of what was discovered yesterday was so powerful, we're ready for the next strike, unlike the first time. It's not going to surprise us, stun us, or floor us. Whenever that cancer makes a move, we'll be ready to make our counterattack. It's going to have to work a lot harder to take you from us now and I suspect it doesn't have the same stamina as you and the thousands of supporters following your story.

So I have to ask, since I wasn't there for most of the day, did anyone ask for your autograph after your television appearance yesterday? I imagined a line of groupies waiting outside of your door hoping to catch a glimpse of Brave Will in his room. The TV station said so many people wanted to see your story, they decided to add the video to their website so people could not only read about you, but see you too.

While I only got to spend a few hours with you tonight, you gave me an extra special gift while I was holding you--my first smile from you. I heard from your grandma and mom that you had been starting to give them out, but so far, it was only a folk tale to me. I needed to see it for myself. So as I held you tonight and you finally caught my eyes, I watched with great delight as that smile slowly grew across your face and stayed there for what seemed like minutes. And you kept doing it until it just tired you out. It was an image that I feared I would never see, but now it is emblazoned in my memory and will be the last thing I picture before I close my eyes and fall asleep...

Be brave
Be strong
We love you!

FRIDAY, OCTOBER 24, 2008

Brave Will,

After such an amazing week, there's really little else to say, so I'll keep things brief. I'm spending the night with you tonight and need to get my sleep. There's a big event planned in your honor tomorrow and I want to be well rested so I can proudly represent you.

We're in a nice holding pattern right now. You must have been in a little pain from your chemo this week because as soon as they gave just a little morphine, your heart rate went back down. Your counts are crashing now, which is to be expected. Next week will be critical for you as you become more and more at risk for infection and illness. We're going to watch for every little sign and make sure that no one with any kind of sickness comes too close because we need to get those counts back up to normal without complications. Once those counts return, we will be able to focus on the next steps. The first step will be to take an official MRI so we can see just how much of that tumor in your brain is left. After that, your doctor is looking to start a third round of treatment. She said that we can only do the really heavy stuff for so long, so she wants to make sure she gets as much of the tumors out of you before we have to start a lower dose of medicine. We had conversations about how a one-year treatment would go and talked about potential delay issues you might have as you get older. Can you believe we are actually talking about this stuff? I certainly can't. I think of the conversations we were having last month and think about how we couldn't look beyond the next day, and now we're talking about six months from now and even kindergarten. I still remain guarded, waiting for the other shoe to drop because we've been whacked so many times over the last few weeks, but maybe it doesn't have to be this way this time.

Maybe, just maybe, we've turned the corner...

Be brave
Be strong
We love you!

SATURDAY, OCTOBER 25, 2008

Brave Will,

I'm going to veer from the normal letter to you today. I spent the day at a fundraiser that some incredible people held in your honor. I had planned on speaking to the huge number of supporters at the event, but couldn't go through with it. It was such a day of celebration and I wasn't sure I would be able to hold it together, so I thought it would be best to just stand and admire.

So, instead of writing only to you tonight, I'd like to write to them and say all the things I wasn't able to say today...

I want to thank anyone who was involved in arranging the fundraiser today. I was simply amazed and incredibly humbled to be standing among people who devoted so much time and effort to our family. The event was flawless and attended by family, friends, colleagues, and people we've never even met, and it was all because of our little Brave Will. I know he has driven people to perform tireless, selfless acts and today was a prime example of what a strong community can do.

I want to thank anyone who was there today who has supported, prayed, thought, donated, visited, called, or written to us. Your actions, no matter how small you may think they are, have a profound impact on our ability to move from day to day throughout this entire ordeal. There is never a "right" thing to do in a situation like this. Tammy and I have felt all along that every individual needs to do what they feel most comfortable doing to support us. Every effort you make on our behalf is appreciated and never will be forgotten.

I want to thank our families, who have taken the strength of family bonds to new limits, whether you're a mom, dad, sister, brother, aunt, uncle, grandparent, or cousin. We have leaned on you time and time again for the past six weeks, yet the weight of our burden has never caused the bonds to falter one bit.

I want to especially thank my sister-in-law Helene. From the minute we learned of Will's diagnosis, she has been our voice and has done things to allow Tammy and me to focus all of our energy on our little Will. I know she knows how much she means to Tammy, but I don't think she truly realizes just how much she means to me.

I want to thank our moms and dads. I know it hasn't been easy seeing your baby boy and baby girl suffer through these last six weeks. However, our ability to deal with this situation is a direct reflection on how well you have prepared Tammy and me to be a mother and father. What we have taken from each one of you, and how we have used it as we have built our own family, has been such a source of strength. We are proud of the life lessons you have taught us and those lessons are helping us clear the hurdles that stand in front of us now.

I want to thank our little boys, Ben and Max. I realize this time has been difficult to understand and I know you probably don't know if you're coming or going every single day. It hurts your mom and dad to know that we haven't been able to be there for you each and every day, but we see just how courageous you have both proven to be, so we know you're taking very good care of yourselves, even in our absence.

Finally, I want to really thank the two people who couldn't stand beside me today.

Will--I know many people have been thanking you for helping to put their own lives into perspective. For me, you have done that and so much more. I am simply a better father, husband, son, brother, friend, and colleague for knowing you. You have shown me the good in so many other people. You have shown me that random strangers can open their hearts and take my breath away with a random act of kindness, as I witnessed time and time again today. You have shown me that little flaws in people are dwarfed by an even bigger heart. Why it took something like this to get me to see that, I'll never know. But since this had to happen, I'm thankful I am wiser from it.

Lastly, I want to thank my wife. There is no way she would ever think of leaving the bedside of her son to be at the event today and that's what makes her so special. I have been the face of our relationship throughout the past few weeks, but she is truly the rock in this partnership. My job is easy by comparison. What she does day in and day out, I can only dream of being capable of and I am in awe of her ability to be the most incredible mother to three of the most incredible little boys every single moment of their lives. It would be impossible to walk along this path we are on alone, and I can't think of anyone else in this world I would want holding my hand to guide us.

I would never wish what we have endured upon anyone. But since this is the path we have been guided down, I feel so lucky to have all of these people standing right beside me. Please don't ever stop doing whatever it is that you have done that has allowed the miracles of this past week to take place. There are simply some things that cannot be easily explained. We still have a long road ahead of us, and your unwavering support will be critical in the times to come.

Thank you all...

Be brave
Be strong
We love you!

MONDAY, OCTOBER 27, 2008

Brave Will,

It's been strange to have things be so stable for the last few days. As they have told us many times, stability is a good thing in the oncology business. So, you've been holding your own as your counts have steadily dropped lower and lower. You just about hit the bottom now and we'll watch over the next few days as things start to climb again. And what do you get as a reward for this? How 'bout another round of chemo!! It doesn't seem like much of a prize for all of your hard work, but we know we've got to keep going after this thing to make sure we obliterate anything that's still up there and in your leg. Your doctor has said she might be too anxious to wait until after round three and may squeak in an MRI before your next round begins sometime next week. I, too, wouldn't mind that peace of mind to know that what they saw in the CAT scan last week was really true.

It's strange--you've been on such a roll for the past week and our family has been floating, but yet your mom and I were saying tonight that we're both afraid. We've been bitten so many times that we're cautiously peeking around every corner unsure of what might be waiting there for you. I guess I just expect at some point that we'll get knocked down again. I hope this doesn't happen and wish every moment that it won't, but the reality of this type of cancer is that it doesn't go quietly, and when it does come back, it's usually pretty mean the second time around. So while your mom and I are ecstatic at the progress you have been making, there's that little piece that can't seem to escape the darkest spaces of our minds. I guess you call what we have "guarded optimism". We'd love to send you through another round of chemo and find out it is pretty much gone--you would certainly be in the medical books if that were the case. But we also know that we can't turn our back on this thing for a minute and rest comfortably. We have to be aware that this battle is far from over.

So I'm going to continue to celebrate your successes and marvel at your bravery and strength. But please don't mind me if I'm looking a little worried sometimes or may be overreacting to some of the smaller stuff that would normally go unnoticed. What can I say, I'm a parent after all, and that's what we do best...we worry about our children.

Be brave
Be strong
We love you!

TUESDAY, OCTOBER 28, 2008

Brave Will,

Can you believe it--snow on October 28th!?! I'm so glad you got to see your first snowfall. Your brothers love playing outside in the snow and I hope one day you'll have lots of opportunities to make snowmen and have a snowball fight with Ben and Max.

So, because of work and class, I didn't get to see you today, which felt a little odd. However, your mom said you are still doing well with everything. Your doctor came to visit and said she is targeting next week to do an MRI and then to follow that right up with your next round of chemotherapy. Once you recover from treatment, you'll probably have some sort of surgery and it will really depend on what they see at that time--will there be something to take out in your brain? Will the tumor in your leg shrink enough to remove it? Those are the things that will need to be decided sometime next month. For now, they just need those counts to start rising again.

Tonight I got to experience a little bit of the new normal. When I got back to the hotel tonight, your mom was waiting for me in the room while grandma watched you back at the hospital. She had dinner waiting and your brothers were in bed "trying" to fall asleep, if you define "trying" as making each other laugh and throwing stuffed animals at each other for nearly two hours. It was such a wonderful sound to hear them giggling in the other room while your mom and I ate together. It's as close as we've come to feeling like a family again in quite some time. The doctors are hopeful that after we get through the next round of treatment, you will be able to spend a few hours here and there with us in the hotel room. A full family of five--can you imagine that finally happening? Just having you here in the room will be such a monumental accomplishment for something we would have dreamed about a month ago. I'll make sure we save a seat for you at the dinner table...

Be brave
Be strong
We love you!

WEDNESDAY, OCTOBER 29, 2008

Brave Will,

As we continue to wait for your counts to rise, your mom decided that today was a day to give back. She and auntie arranged for sandwiches, salads, and snacks to be brought in for all of the doctors and nurses that have been by our side since day one. It was our way of saying thank you for all of the hard work and tremendous care they have given you over the past six weeks. You know what your mom says, "When in need, we feed." It seems like such a small gesture compared to what they have done for us. I honestly don't know how they are able to do this day in and day out. We are simply one of many situations they stand in front of daily, and yet they keep coming back every single day. They have truly helped us make the best of a bad situation with grace and compassion.

We continue our march down that path but do so knowing that the eyes and minds of many brilliant professionals are doing everything in their power to make you a success story.

Be brave
Be strong
We love you!

THURSDAY, OCTOBER 30, 2008

Brave Will,

You know what I'm struggling with tonight? I thought I was struggling with the fact that I didn't know what to write tonight. Then I realized that it's not that I don't know what to write, it's that I don't get to spend enough time with you to truly know how things are going from day to day so that I can tell you about it each night. It's crazy--a couple of weeks ago, I was sad because I never got to see your brothers. Your mom and I made some changes to allow us to see your brothers nearly every day. Unfortunately, that has meant that I only get to see you for an hour or so a day, and now that's making me sad. I'll tell you Will, there's just no pleasing me...

When I don't get to see you as much, I have to ask your mom all kinds of questions about how your day went, what the doctors said, and what the next steps are. She answers all of my questions, but the amount of information is so difficult to process that I end up spending my nights trying to sort it all out in my head and end up with a lot more questions. Like today, your mom said you were in a lot of pain because of the sores in your mouth from chemo. So what does that mean? Did they put you back on the morphine simply because of the sores? Will you come off of it as soon as the sores go away? When do the sores go away? I miss being able to sit beside you all day as the doctors and nurses come in. You'll soon learn that I'm the type of person that needs to know all of the information, all the facts. When I don't get all of that, I feel left out like I'm missing something. Unfortunately, in this situation, there's really not much I or your mom can do about it. Fortunately, you're not the type to hold a grudge, it appears. So when all is said and done, I'm hoping you don't hold this against me. Besides, your mom spends enough time by your side for the both of us, and she's got an awful lot of love inside of her to make up for my absence.

So tomorrow, I'm hoping to spend a little more time with you. We're going to take Ben and Max trick-or-treating. They're only just a tiny bit excited about going out and getting tons of candy! Can't wait to be able to take you out next year--can we make sure that happens? At any rate, after that, I'm gonna crash at your place, if you don't mind. We'll catch up a little bit--I'll tell you all about trick-or-treating, the World Series, and whatever else you might want to know...

Be brave
Be strong
We love you!

FRIDAY, OCTOBER 31, 2008

Brave Will,

Happy Halloween, little buddy. I'm not sure that your formula and TPN are as sweet as a Snickers bar or M&M's, but at this point, we'd much rather see you get a bottle down instead of a Milky Way. Your mom and I were able to take your brothers out trick-or-treating. In fact, while you stayed with grandma and papa, your mom surprised Ben at his school today and was able to see the big Halloween parade. Ben was dressed as a yellow Transformer and Max was a dragon. I didn't

get to see you in costume today, but I understand you were dressed as a brain surgeon, which is fitting. I think the nurses were calling you Dr. McDreamy, you handsome stud.

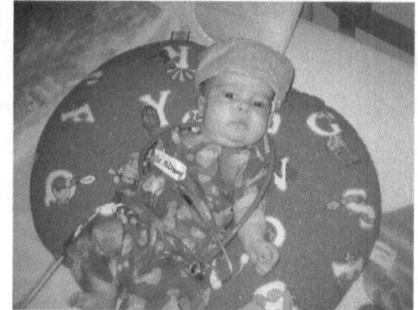

When I got to the room tonight, I was thrilled to see you were wide awake (watching football, naturally). We had some nice awake time together before you finally drifted off. You appear to be in less pain than you were yesterday so maybe we can get you back off the morphine this weekend. The sores in your mouth must be getting better too since you were willing to drink from the bottle and use your pacifier.

So, you know you've hit the big time when you have a website with your own web address. All the big stars have one. So I'm pleased to let you know that we've developed a special website just for you: www.bravewill.com. I'm still going to use this site to write my letters to you and I hope that your supporters will continue to leave you notes here as well. However, on the other site, we can show some more pictures of you, share some video, post information about fundraisers that people are holding in your name, and also let people have a chance to get some Brave Will gear that some have been asking about. You need to be a pretty special someone to have a dot com address name after you...and I think you've earned it.

Be brave
Be strong
We love you!

SUNDAY, NOVEMBER 02, 2008

Brave Will,

It was great spending time with you this weekend. We got to spend the night together on Friday and then hung out a lot on Saturday and Sunday. There's one thing that is clear--you are acting more and more like a 3 1/2 month old baby. If someone were to walk in your room, they probably wouldn't even be able to tell you were sick (outside of those tubes all around you). Today alone, you had some great belly time and spent some time in your baby swing--very normal baby activities. All that activity tired you out, as expected. Fortunately for you, I was up for taking a nap with you and let you sleep on me while I dozed off. Must've been the time change...

So this is a pretty big week for you, me, and your mom. Your counts have started to climb and it looks like they're going to take a picture of your head on Thursday. I'll probably talk more about this as it gets closer, but I can tell you, your mom and I are really nervous about this. On one hand, we need that picture to confirm what the doctors saw a couple of weeks ago--that the tumor in your head has reduced in size. On the other hand, we could find that it could have grown back in the last two weeks. You know, like always, that your mom and I are staying very positive about what the outcome will be and honestly, there's not a lot of use in thinking too much about this now. Regardless of the outcome, we will deal with whatever we see in the MRI. That being said, I've told you before, your mom and I like to worry because it's what we do best, and right now, we feel worried...

As we hit the 50-day mark of our stay at the hospital, we can't help but think about how much we're ready to put this all behind us and move on all together as a family. We know we can't do that...not yet--there's still too much work left to be done. Yet every now and again, you just hit a rut where you want to be in someone else's life instead of where we are at. The rut doesn't last for too long, thankfully, but it does drain a lot of the energy out of you. Here's hoping that the good news continues this week and gives us the energy to pull through with whatever comes our way next.

Be brave
Be strong
We love you!

MONDAY, NOVEMBER 03, 2008

Brave Will,

I wasn't sure I was going to write tonight because I wasn't quite sure what to say to you. I guess I'm still in that rut I talked about yesterday, and didn't want that mood to be reflected in my letter to you. Then I read Father Ken's posting on your guestbook tonight and I realized the importance of the words he used: "stay in the moment". Very good advice from a very wise man...

I know I'm extremely nervous about your coming MRI, and your mom and I talked tonight about what we're expecting when we hear about the results--what will we do if it's good news and what we will do if it's bad news. But there's no point in wasting energy on that now. Your mom and I need to stay in the moment and enjoy you on Tuesday, enjoy you on Wednesday, and enjoy you on Thursday just like we've been doing for the past 5 days. Looking too far ahead puts us in such a defenseless position. We know we can control how we feel tomorrow and tomorrow only, so that's what I need to focus my attention on.

So I promise I'm not going to dwell on what could happen later this week and just do what your mom and I said we would do all along--just appreciate each and every day we get to spend with you and stay in the moment...

Be brave
Be strong
We love you!

TUESDAY, NOVEMBER 04, 2008

Brave Will,

Just a quick medical update tonight since I haven't really talked too much about this over the past couple of days. I got to the hotel late tonight so I didn't get a chance to see you at the hospital today. Your mom, in her best impression of a nurse, gave me an update on everything that happened today. Your counts have slowly but surely climbed up to where they need to be. By the end of the week, you should be right where the doctors need you to be.

The doctors have also been watching your feeding very closely. Even though you have been starting to feel a little better this week, you are still not eating a lot for a little baby. And when you do eat, you're having a hard time keeping the food in your belly. Today, you took a field trip in the hospital to get a test where they had you take a special drink and then watched on a monitor how the food traveled from your mouth to your belly. They didn't notice anything too alarming but thought we might need to add a little something extra to your formula to make it a little thicker. You're not ready for solid food quite yet, so hopefully the thicker formula will successfully stay in your belly. If you don't like the outfits your mother dresses you in, there are easier ways to get changed instead of throwing up over everything!

It's yet another small hurdle that we've grown accustomed to dealing with on a regular basis. These little tests, which two years ago would have crippled us with anxiety, barely go by with much attention at all. It's those much bigger hurdles that we're still learning how to clear.

Anxiety has certainly taken on a new life in your mom and me. I remember about four years ago when your brother Ben got tubes in his ears. We were so scared to let the doctors take him to the operating room and out of our arms. Less than ten really long minutes (it felt like two hours), it was over. Now, anxiety is sending you in for two hours of brain surgery; anxiety is having a shunt put in your head when the surgeons say you aren't well enough for surgery; anxiety is waiting for the results of an MRI to see what the future holds for you. I hope that one day we'll be "fortunate" to just send you in to have tubes put in your ears. That's a kind of anxiety I would gladly welcome once again...

Be brave
Be strong
We love you!

Brave Will,

A family. Tonight, we were finally a family and it felt so incredible. There were no tubes, no medicines, no nurses, no beeps, no painkillers, no doctors, no antibiotics. It was just you, me, your mom, Ben and Max. We got to spend four hours all together in the hotel room and all had dinner together. It was crazy, noisy, and chaotic--exactly what we wanted it to be. I'm hopeful this will be the first of many nights to come while we spend our time here, and eventually this will become part of everyday life when we move into our new home. Will, I'd forgotten what this all felt like and I realized I missed it...a lot. I'm not going to lie to you, it definitely made saying goodbye to you and your mom tonight that much harder. But I can get used to it if it means we can spend more time outside the walls of the hospital.

It's good thing you can't eat solid food because the way you were sucking down bottles today, you would have eaten every last bit of our dinner tonight. Apparently, the doctors found the missing ingredient in your formula because we haven't seen you eat this well since we first arrived at the hospital. This is what we're used to seeing with a 3-month old baby and it makes your mom and me so happy to be able to feed you. There's just so little that we can do to make you feel better--making sure you're not hungry is one of those things that we will always be there to help you with.

So tomorrow is a pretty big day. In the afternoon, they'll put you asleep for a couple of hours so they can take pictures of your head, leg, and wherever else they want to examine. They want to take as many pictures as possible so they can see how things look compared to what they saw back in September. They know from the CAT scan that things looked pretty good a couple of weeks ago. However, this is the "official" picture. Will things be better than two weeks ago or worse? If they are worse, will the picture still be better than what they saw in September? More importantly, what does this all mean for you? As you can tell, I've got lots of questions rattling around upstairs in my head. I just know that what we hopefully find out tomorrow will dictate where we go next and it scares the heck out of me. I'm ready for whatever path we're headed down and I've thought about all of the possibilities, but obviously, there are certain outcomes that your mom and I are hoping to hear. Whatever your pictures show, my little friend, don't forget for even a moment that your mom and I are standing right beside you no matter what happens next. We'll get through tomorrow and the next day and the next, just like we've gotten through the past 55 days.

But tomorrow is definitely going to be one of the most important ones that will probably not soon forget...

Be brave
Be strong
We love you!

THURSDAY, NOVEMBER 06, 2008

Brave Will,

You're about to go in for your MRI and your mom and I are so happy that you are continuing to hold onto hope.

Be brave
Be strong
We love you!

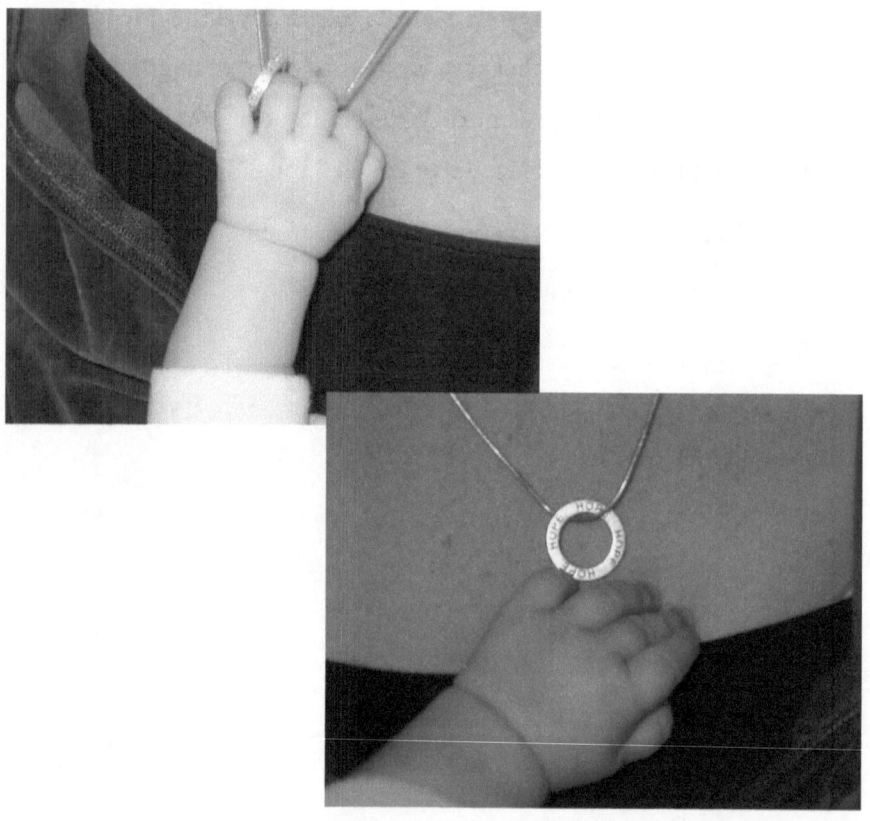

THURSDAY, NOVEMBER 06, 2008

Brave Will,

Okay, so where do we start tonight? I guess I'll begin by saying that so far, and "unofficially", you did very well on your tests today! The doctors we spoke to all said the same thing--that they need to get the official word from a person who reads MRI pictures for a living. However, in their professional opinions as doctors who look at these pictures every day, when they looked at the MRI of your head, they are having a difficult time finding any resemblance of a tumor there. Can you believe I just said that?? What they suspected two weeks ago was again proven to be the case. Now, a little word of caution before we all get even more excited (if that's possible)--cancer cells are tricky things. Even when tumors go away, little microscopic cells can still remain there and can start growing again to become tumors. There is still a possibility of this happening. But here's the good news--we're not stopping. We're going to keep treating you as if that tumor was still there so that any cells that might be trying to grow will continue to melt away.

Now, as for the leg...there's still something there, which we expected. We have been able to see that there is something still hanging around your right leg, so we weren't surprised. But once again, what they saw in September versus what they saw today was definitely better. The doctors still want the official word from the radiologist tomorrow to fully comprehend what they saw, but there's no question progress has been made. But unlike the head, there's still some immediate work that will need to be done. They'll need to figure out how to get that tumor out of your leg and have to determine where it resides--muscle or bone. This will likely mean more surgery for you at some point, but not until after another round of the ocean waves first to see if we can't make that mass a little smaller.

So all told, we're pretty happy with what we heard. We still keep that guarded optimism, and know we want the official word tomorrow, but there's no question this was about the best news we could have gotten today. Still, we know this isn't close to the end and there are lots left to be done, but my little friend, we are headed in the right direction.

It looks like we'll get a little break this weekend. Your counts are high enough and your next round won't begin until Monday, so they'll let you take some leaves-of-absence this weekend. We've got big plans, little man, big plans. You know what's a little strange? You're nearly four months old and today was probably the healthiest day of your life. There were no medicines in you, tumors had begun to wash away, and you have been eating more than you have since we have been here. How good it must feel right now--we're so glad we were able to enjoy it with you. I just know that there are even bigger, better, healthier days ahead for you.

I can feel that faith and hope that so many have been holding onto for the last two months. I can feel it driving us forward, lifting us higher, and keeping us going as we move into our next phase, whatever that may be. No matter what happens from here, for the better and even the worse, Brave Will, you are truly our little miracle baby.

Be brave
Be strong
We love you!

SATURDAY, NOVEMBER 08, 2008

Brave Will,

So our weekend pass ended up getting cut a little short. We spoke at length with your doctor this morning and she said as much as she would like to give us another day to hang with the whole family tomorrow, she just doesn't want to wait another day to start round three of the ocean waves. We were thankful that we got to enjoy having you at the hotel again for dinner last night and then, for the first time in two months, you got to leave the Albany area with all of us today. We took you up to the new house to show you where your room is going to be when it is finished. You seemed to enjoy the space and I think your brothers are coming to the realization that you have the biggest room even though they got to pick their rooms out first. I don't know how you did it, but you managed to sell them both on the idea of taking smaller rooms--well done, little man. After visiting the house, we had a nice dinner out at Friendly's and then it was back to the hospital with your mom, where you'll now be for a few weeks. I guess, after talking to the doctor, that we realized why we are here. Sure family time is nice and necessary, but the only reason we are down here is to make sure you get better and if that means starting your next round of treatment a day earlier than we planned, then so be it. You are our purpose, our job and it's a job that we don't take lightly.

I got to see the scans that they took on Friday and was able to compare them to the ones that were taken on September 14th. I was absolutely stunned when I saw the images of your brain. On 9/14, there was this huge mass just sitting in the back of your brain resting against the "command center" of your entire body. In the scans that they took

Thursday, there is literally nothing visible in that area. Still doesn't mean that the cells are gone entirely, but there is definitely nothing as large and as dangerous as what you had then. There are a couple of small spots elsewhere that your doctor wants to keep an eye on. It's difficult to say if they are anything at all, but she is not taking any chances. Hopefully, if they are related, the next round will wipe those out as well. After all, you have conquered much bigger mountains than that already.

Your leg scans are certainly a different story. Again, by comparison, the area of the tumor is definitely smaller now, so the good news is that the chemo is affecting that area somewhat. However, the scans still show two areas of muscle being affected as well as bone. This is what needs to be attacked now. While it's hard to say if the leg was the primary location of your cancer, it's pretty safe to say that this area is far more advanced than the area in your head. The doctors would like to do some more tests in the near future to see how much of what they still see in the muscle is still alive and thriving and how much of it is now just dead tissue and cells. In addition, they're going to need to test your bones to make sure that the bad cells aren't traveling in your bone marrow to other locations. This was something they were going to do the first week we were here, but your mom and I decided not to have that procedure done because you had been through so much already and it wouldn't have affected your treatment at all. However, now we want the conclusive proof of how this cancer is getting around your body.

While you are getting your third round of the ocean waves, your doctor will be sending your MRI's to surgeons around the northeast. She will be looking for the perfect person that has the best skills to go into your tiny little leg and try to remove what might still be there after we finish round three. There is a strong likelihood that this will mean that you, your mom, and I will have to leave your brothers for a few days to travel to a different city to talk to doctors and eventually have surgery. It's not a shock--we pretty much expected this would have to happen at some point. I think by having your brothers spend more time with us in the hotel has been a good thing. When we have to take these little trips, they'll better understand why we have to go and know that we are doing what is best for you. They also know that they'll be right back with us as soon as we return.

We're kind of in a strange spot right now. We managed to get past the first two months, which few expected you would be able to do. We've seen tremendous improvement in your condition, yet we know we're far from safe and still have so far to go to feel any kind of security. But now we're at that point where we have to look ahead a little bit. We have to think about the next steps of your treatment. We have to be cognizant of how this disease works and how it can be defeated. There's just so many factors that go into play and so many pieces that have to align perfectly to make this work. So far, things have fallen into place better than we could have imagined. As we begin the next stage of treatment, the next phase of potential recovery, and the next path of the journey, I can't help but wonder just where things are headed next and I look forward, not with fear, but with cautious optimism, to finding out...

Be brave
Be strong
We love you!

SUNDAY, NOVEMBER 09, 2008

Brave Will,

I was pretty busy with your brothers today so I didn't get to see you for that long. We got up early and ran a few errands and then we got a chance to visit the state museum. They had a lot of fun seeing all of the cool things there and it was great to spend so much time with them today. Of course, because your weekend pass got cut a little short, it meant that we didn't get to have you there with us. However, your mom said you were busy starting your next round of the ocean waves. Today, you got the ocean water and yellow flower. It's strange how relaxed we are this time around. I mean, after all, this is only the third time you've received chemotherapy, yet we feel like old veterans at this thing. The good news is that the nurses and doctors are learning a little more each time they use this treatment plan, and therefore, we're again hoping for limited side effects. There was only just a little swelling today and at least while I was there, when you woke up, you eagerly devoured an entire bottle. If you can keep this up, then we'll be able to remove the nutritional supplement they have been giving you.

Your mom is also going to be working a lot on your movement. Because you have been so sick, you've spent so much of your days in bed on your back. As a result, the muscles in your neck need to develop more so that you can begin to hold your head up and turn your head on your own. These actions were basically unable to be done for almost two months because we were so afraid to move you. Now that things have improved all over, we're going to give you more to do--belly time, sitting you up, time in your swing, and holding you more and more when we feed you. The doctor said these things are going to be critical in your ability to "catch up" to other babies your age.

All this activity for you is a little bittersweet. It was so nice to see you look and feel so healthy for the past few days. You were alert, smiling, cooing, and content. We know this can't last as these medicines invade your body. But again, we remind ourselves that the reason we are here is to make you better and while those days of healthiness are nice, we need to take every step to ensure that all of your days are healthy, not just a few here and there.

Be brave
Be strong
We love you!

MONDAY, NOVEMBER 10, 2008

Brave Will,

Well my first effort at writing to you tonight got wiped out by a technical error (I hate technology sometimes!). So I don't know that I'll be able to say things the same way I really wanted to, but I'll give it another shot.

Round three, day two is in the books and I'm happy to hear things are going well so far. You also passed a hearing test today, which is critical because one of the chemo drugs you receive does have a risk of leading to hearing lost. It's good to know you can still hear those ocean waves that we play for you when you receive treatment.

Unfortunately, today was a long day for me and I didn't get a chance to see you. The good news is that I will be able to spend all day with you tomorrow. Your mom said that you are still smiling a lot, so I'm hoping you've got some saved up for me tomorrow. I know that this won't last for too much longer before you start to feel yucky again, so I'm going to soak it in for as long as possible.

I'm feeling pretty sad for another reason today. Your mom and I read about another little boy today who has the same type of tumor that you have. His name is Jonathan and his dad has posted in your guestbook before and created a website that I have linked from your Brave Will website. At any rate, Jonathan had an MRI on Saturday and they found out today that while Jonathan's original tumor is still gone, another one has grown in his brain and they don't believe that surgery can be done. I felt absolutely devastated to hear this. I know how joyful it is to hear that the tumors have melted away and I can imagine the sorrow his mom and dad must feel knowing that this disease has found another way back. I doubt that Jonathan's mom and dad ever felt like they were in the clear with this, just as your mom and I never feel that way. But still, you get these thoughts from time to time that maybe your son might just beat the dismal odds that are associated with this type of cancer--an anomaly to the statistics, as your mom likes to say. I just wonder how you can stop this thing--how did those "anomalies" do it and survive? This doesn't mean that Jonathan won't have eventual success, or that we're destined for bad news in the future. It just shows how difficult this is really going to be. It just means that we'll be incapable of any kind of safety or relief for a long, long time. Even in those times of joy, I'm sure I'll still be looking over my shoulder.

I'll go to bed tonight thinking of you like I always do. But tonight I'll be thinking of Jonathan too and his mom and dad. I hope that whatever path their recent news takes them down now will be filled with the same wisdom, support, and love that we have been so fortunate to have for the past two months. I wish for them renewed hope as their journey takes a new turn.

Be brave
Be strong
We love you!

TUESDAY, NOVEMBER 11, 2008

Brave Will,

Just a great day with you today, a great day. I haven't been able to spend so much time with you in quite a while, so I feel so rejuvenated having been around you all day. You certainly haven't started feeling the effects of the chemotherapy yet as you were all smiles today. It seemed like if you weren't sleeping or eating, you were smiling, and I loved every minute of it. There was even a time today that you were being fussy with your mom so she handed you back off to me and you settled right in and gave me the biggest grin like you knew you'd gotten rid of the "old lady".

You know you are having a good day when the neurosurgeon comes into the room and tells you there's no work left for him in your head anymore and that his services just aren't needed at this time. I apologized to him for keeping him unemployed. I don't care how many times I hear someone tell us that things look clear in your head--I never get tired of it. I almost asked him to say it to your mom and I a second time just so we could hear it one more time but I figured he had better things to do with his time.

Your tests continued today and this one was a little more painful than your hearing test yesterday. Today they had to test your cerebral spine fluid (CSF). The way they test is by putting a small needle in the shunt that is in the back of your head. Your mom and I stood out in the hall for that one but we heard you loud and clear that this was not a test you want to take again anytime soon. At any rate, the shunt that they tapped contains a small little sack that holds the fluid that circulates around your brain. When they take that fluid out and run some tests on it, they can determine if the fluid contains cancerous cells. This will help the doctors determine if, despite the fact that the tumor has shrunk, there are still some cancerous cells floating around your brain and spine. It won't change your treatment at all because we are still going forward with the ocean waves regardless, but it does give us a bigger picture of what challenges might still remain in your brain. We should hear about the results later in the week.

I ended my day with you by meeting with your doctor while you slept in my arms. It was great to spend a while with her and I asked lots of questions about you. I often only get to ask questions through your mom because I'm usually at work when the doctors stop in to see you. So today, I was able to grill her with everything that I had been rolling around in my head. She was so patient with me, answering all of my questions, thinking about different paths we might take in our next round, and offering a lot of suggestions for helping you to "catch up" in your development. I didn't walk away with any more hope, nor any more desperation, and I didn't expect to. I simply walked away knowing that we have a short term plan, we have lots of decisions to continue to make, and lots of options to explore as we get beyond round three. It seemed like the first two months were built around "we need to do this, or else..." Now I feel like we can make some rational decisions, as uncharted as they may be for all of us. It also means the decisions will be harder because the choices will all sound like reasonable options. Nevertheless, I would never turn down the chance to continue to make decisions on your behalf. The fact that we are still in a position to have to make choices is far better than any outcome we, and the doctors, could have hoped for at this point in your life.

Be brave
Be strong
We love you!

WEDNESDAY, NOVEMBER 12, 2008

Brave Will,

And with the last drop of desert sunset flowing into your body, round three of the ocean waves has come to an end. That's the easy part...and now we wait. Inevitably, once again, your counts will plummet in about a week and we'll need to again be cognizant of potential infections and related fevers. That's always the nervous part. Having toxic medicines running throughout your body for four days-- not a problem; getting a slight 100 degree temperature--big problem. Strange how that works...

The doctor told us that a goal is to try to keep you off of the nutritional supplement (TPN) as this can be a conduit for infection and so far we've been able to dodge that bullet. However, keeping you on this even longer is constantly leaving that door open, so we're going to try and bulk you up through your feedings. We met with a nutritionist who is going to help us add more calories to your bottle and then in a couple of weeks, we'll give you a shot at cereal. If you manage to take to all of this, then the TPN can go away.

I guess we'll all be watching your counts closely for the next two weeks. We're hoping that they'll climb just in time to allow you to join the whole family for Thanksgiving. It's going to be close, but if you're able to pass the desert sunset as quickly as you did last round, you might have a shot. It's generally about a two week process for your counts to drop and then build back up, so that puts us right on the doorstep of Thanksgiving if all goes perfectly (does it ever?). But as Father Ken told us yesterday, even if you can't be with us while we eat, it won't matter because every day that we have you here with us is Thanksgiving. Besides, if you're still stuck in bed, it gives me a place to go crash once the turkey coma kicks in...make room for daddy!

Be brave
Be strong
We love you!

FRIDAY, NOVEMBER 14, 2008

Brave Will,

Happy 4-month birthday! You sure were chatty tonight telling me all about your big day. That infectious smile coupled with your little cooing sounds was the perfect pick-me-up for the end of the week. Despite it being your 1/3 birthday, your mom still hasn't taken it easy on you in her quest to turn you into Hercules. In one short week, she's managed to turn your room into a children's version of Gold's Gym. Every morning, she puts you through workout circuits--a little swing time, followed by 10 minutes of belly time, then some time in the bouncy seat, followed by laps around the C7 wing strapped to mom in the Baby Bjorn. I'm not even sure people training for the triathlon have it as hard as you do. But it's starting to have some good effects. You're definitely getting more strength in your little body and hopefully soon, you'll build up those neck muscles to allow you to lift your head up all on your own.

More good news today. The results of the test that you took earlier this week came back clean. They looked at your cerebrospinal fluid and found no indications of cancerous cells that may be traveling throughout your brain and spine. Another passing grade, my little man! This was a big one because it again confirmed what the MRIs showed us last week--no visible sign of the brain tumor. Additionally, it also indicates that there are no remnant cells lingering upstairs either. So this is a great sign and means we have to keep working hard to make sure we keep those nasty cells out of there now that the area is clean. I am so thrilled by the news but still need to keep that guarded optimism that I've told you about. I just don't want to get knocked as low as we did before, so the only way to do that is to keep myself closer to the ground. So I may be all smiles and laughs, and be as upbeat as I have been for two months, but please know, it's going to take a lot longer to heal some of the pains that have built inside of me. Like those tumors inside of you, the pains I have likely won't easily subside, and may linger for quite some time. I'll work on mine as long as you continue to work on yours.

Be brave
Be strong
We love you!

SUNDAY, NOVEMBER 16, 2008

Brave Will,

Well, you must be doing something right to get all of these special privileges that you got this weekend. First, on Saturday, you again got to take a field trip. With your counts expected to take a dip very soon, we wanted to have one more shot with you outside of the hospital. Your brothers were spending time this weekend with grandparents, aunts, uncles, and cousins, so it was just the three of us. Your mom and I got about five hours of "freedom" with you--always

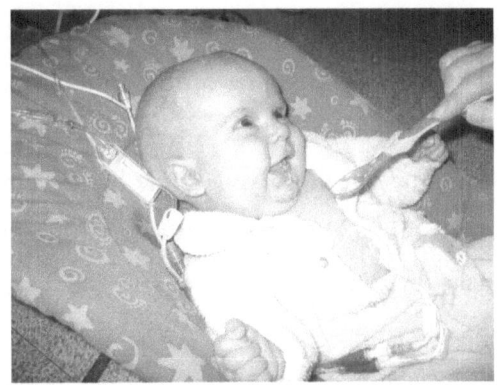

special time...I loved looking at your eyes as we stepped outside and you felt the fresh air. It must feel so incredible to have the air run through your body--I guess I totally take for granted something so simple that you've barely gotten a chance to experience.

Then, the best privilege of the past weekend was the newest addition to your menu. Your mom was able to feed you solid food for the first time. You obviously enjoyed it, much more than you've been enjoying your formula. You welcomed the new addition to your diet and gummed it down graciously. We're in a tough spot with this feeding thing. We've gotten you to keep your formula down for most of the past week or so. However, it's still not enough to keep your weight up. So now, with the effects of chemo settling in, you're even less likely to want to eat, formula or solid food. As a result, with your weight dropping each day since Thursday, the doctors had no choice but to put you back on the TPN to supplement your nutrition. We're still going to keep going with the food and formula, and as much as we would like this to be enough, we want and need you to remain heavy and healthy over the next couple of weeks when the effects of the ocean waves really start to take its toll. So the TPN is really a necessity at this point. But that is not going to deter us from one of the few things that we are able to do for you.

Beyond the eating issues, you also developed a really bad rash this weekend on your chest. It's difficult to say what caused it, but the doctors didn't waste any time putting you on antibiotics to make sure it didn't become anything serious. Fortunately, it didn't seem to dampen your spirits too much as you were as smiley and talkative as ever. I just love how infectious your smile has become. Even when you wake up out of sound sleep or seem to be a little fussy, as soon as I am able to make eye contact with you or you hear my voice, that smile just spreads across your face. It's so awesome to see that you really know my face and my voice. I guess I had forgotten how wonderful that felt when this happened with your older brothers. Thank you for reminding me again about those little things that can bring so much joy.

Keep smiling, my little friend...

Be brave
Be strong
We love you!

MONDAY, NOVEMBER 17, 2008

Brave Will,

I was just about to call it a night but checked my e-mail and saw something that I just had to share with you.

Your story has definitely hit the ends of the Earth. Our good friend Dave is currently working this month in Antarctica and he e-mailed me some pictures that he took. He put one of your bracelets along with a bracelet for his son Connor and placed them on the pole that marks the geographic South Pole, the southernmost point on the entire planet.

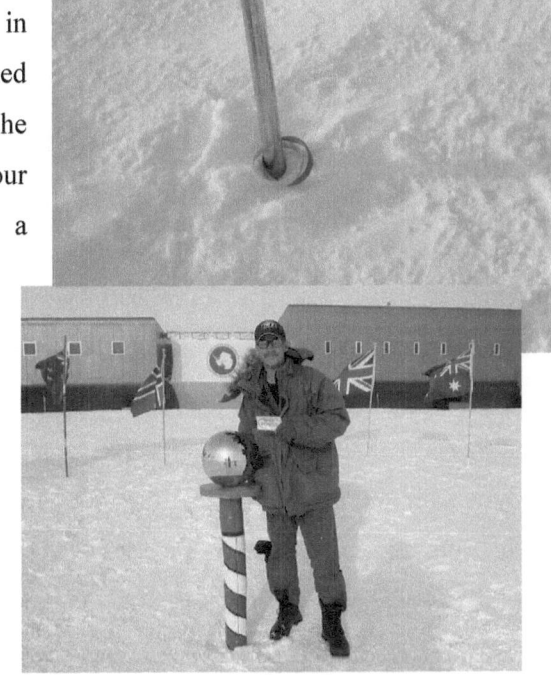

I'm convinced now--your story will eventually reach every continent on Earth...

Be brave
Be strong
We love you!

TUESDAY, NOVEMBER 18, 2008

Brave Will,

Well, as expected, you've definitely hit the bottom this week. Your counts plummeted yesterday and you've been unable to keep any food or formula down. After seeing you so "alive" the past week or so, it's difficult to see you like this. You've been sleeping most of the day, which is probably the best thing for you right now. I was able to coax a couple of smiles out of you when I came to see tonight--thanks for that--but I could tell your heart wasn't really into it.

So for now, we'll wait patiently as we wait for the counts to rise. We're hopeful, and optimistic that your counts will be back to normal by next Thursday. I guess if there is any consolation, when you're at your lowest during the effects of the chemotherapy, it means that the medicine is doing its job. It's hammering away at all of those nasty cancer cells and hopefully driving them away. I'm hoping that they are finding those cells that are still harming your leg and hoping that if anything is trying to come back in your brain, they are being washed away by the medicine.

So sleep well tonight, my little friend, and let's start the quick road to recovery from this most recent round of ocean waves...

Be brave
Be strong
We love you!

Brave Will,

Apparently, your brother Max is missing you so much, he's decided to join you at Albany Med tomorrow. That's right, you're getting a floormate on C7 tomorrow. We found out last week that Max needs to have his tonsils and adenoids out. They do surgery at AMC on Thursdays, so they were able to squeeze him in. He's been having a lot of issues sleeping at night because of breathing problems, so this should make him feel much better. So tomorrow night, your mom and I will both be sleeping at the hospital, one of us with you, the other with Max. The nurses on the floor can't wait to take care of another little Hladun boy--I wonder if they know that he's probably going to give them more of a run for their money than you would ever dream of. Max isn't really sure what's happening tomorrow but he heard there is "happy" involved (his word for ice cream), so he's all in.

Funny that before this all happened, we would have been so nervous to have Max go through this tomorrow. Now, it's barely raised our pulse. Heck buddy, if you can handle brain surgery and chemotherapy, I'm pretty sure your older brother will be able to take a little sore throat after his surgery. I can't wait for a day when those now minor concerns can become big to your mom and me once again. I think I liked getting nervous about the little things a lot more than dealing with these enormous, incomprehensible moments that you are facing each and every day. Maybe one day, you'll "just" need to have your tonsils out too.

So we'll have two Hladun boys recovering tomorrow. Your brother will be in the hospital for less than a day, and then should be back to normal by next week. We're hoping for a similar outcome for you over the next week. You've been at rock bottom for a couple of days now and have been so sick, we can't wait to see you back to your alert self with the endless smiles. The spotlight may shift to Max for just a brief time tomorrow, but know that your complete recovery will never drift from the forefront of our minds.

Be brave
Be strong
We love you!

THURSDAY, NOVEMBER 20, 2008

Brave Will,

Wow, what a crazy day! Your brother Max had a successful surgery today to remove his tonsils and adenoids. He's been happily enjoying the benefits of the arduous task he went through today. So far, he's managed to gobble down six popsicles, an ice cream cup, cup of jello, peaches, pears, and about five glasses of juice. Yes, Max seems to be pulling through surgery just fine. Even your brother Ben got in on the action and was at the doctor's today, diagnosed with impetigo. As a result, he was pretty much quarantined from both of you today. He's spending the night at the hotel with grandma, while your mom and I spend the night with you and Max.

Your mom and I have been bouncing around like pinballs between your room and Max's room down the hall. Your mom is trying to get your brother asleep now, but he's having a hard time sleeping in the strange place that you would probably call home. I also think he's in a little more pain than he's letting on.

You, on the other hand, continue to sleep and sleep. If it was possible, your counts actually dropped even lower today. You're just so unhappy right now. Because the great days washed away my memories of last month, I've forgotten how bad things get when you're down in the dumps like you are right now. There's nary a smile to be found on that sad face of yours. The morphine that they have to give you to deal with the pain from the sores in your mouth sends your eyes off to a whole different world that it's hard to get you to make eye contact with me. When you are awake, it's really not a pleasant time for you, so it's just easier to let you sleep. Unfortunately, this means that you aren't eating at all, which you know is important to your mom and I.

At least we know this can't last forever. Another day or two of this and things should start to rebound for you. Don't wait too much longer for this--I'm ready to have that little baby boy that I was gushing over last week back again.

Be brave
Be strong
We love you!

SUNDAY, NOVEMBER 23, 2008

(Letter from Mom)

Hello my sweet baby boy,

Sorry it has been so long since I have written to you. When you are older and read your letters please know that all the times Daddy was writing to you I was lying by your side whispering in your ear.

Today is our first full day together since Wednesday. Mommy needed to be with Max for his surgery. He decided to play all night, (do you remember him sneaking in your room to wake you and Daddy?), and so I needed sleep on Friday. I am thrilled to be back with you again today, yet sad that I am not with Max nursing him back to health. Your counts are still low buddy, but you have begun sucking on your binky again and took a few sips of formula so I am hoping you will be bouncing back soon.

While I know you are feeling better than when we first arrived 10 weeks ago, you look so sick to me. Your beautiful eyelashes are falling out, your eyebrows are getting thin, and you are losing your hair. When the doctors said you would lose your hair, Daddy and I giggled thinking you were bald already. Yet, now I realize that it is a different type of bald and I hate having another reminder of what you are going through. Someone that Daddy works with sent a necklace with a poem on it:

What Cancer Cannot Do...

It cannot

invade the soul

surpress memories

kill friendship

destroy peace

conquer the spirit

shatter hope

cripple love

corrode faith

steal eternal life

silence courage

I promise buddy to not allow Cancer to damage our whole family. I won't let what you are going through be in vain. I love you so much sweetie and am so sorry for what you must endure.

Be brave
Be strong
We love you!

SUNDAY, NOVEMBER 23, 2008

Brave Will,

Slowly but surely, you're starting to feel a little better. I couldn't really tell this morning. Your mom said last night was pretty rough as those nasty sores in your mouth worsened and caused a lot of pain for you. However, as the day went on, I noticed those big eyes widen and observe; I noticed the corners of your mouth attempt to curl up in a smile and try ever so hard to form one; I noticed you sucking on your pacifier and twice take a bottle and finally drank some formula for the first time since Wednesday; I noticed you starting to talk again, telling us how you've really felt; and I noticed my little baby boy, once again feeling like a little baby boy.

Those counts are still really low, but they are rising, and I'm certain we'll hear that they are even higher tomorrow. On top of that you did something really important tonight. Normally, when you lay in bed you roll your head to one side until your mom or I move you to look a different way. However, today when I was talking to you and your eyes were looking the other way, you turned your head all on your own so you could look at me. The littlest thing brought me so much joy, buddy. It showed me that you are still making those developmental steps and that the strength you so desperately need is there. I'm certain as soon as your counts are close to normal, your mom will have you back in training so that strength can continue to grow.

We have passed ten weeks that we have been at the hospital--it feels like we've been there a lot longer. When I look at you, I have to remember that you are just four months old because there are times that you feel so much older to me, like this ordeal has aged you much faster than your age indicates. So when you do little things like moving your head on your own, it snaps me back to the reality that you are still only a little baby, and despite all that you have been through, have so many milestones to reach and so many things left to accomplish.

Be brave
Be strong
We love you!

MONDAY, NOVEMBER 24, 2008

Brave Will,

Today was one of those days that makes sure you are reminded that this little roller coaster ride we are on is far from over. There was nothing that happened today that put you in grave danger, but there were some things that definitely knocked us back a few steps. It's probably not a bad thing that this reminded us never to get too comfortable (if that's at all possible) and that we constantly have to be on alert, even when we think things are okay.

The main problem today is that the central line that they use to deliver medicines (called a Hickman) broke. Since it is surgically placed in your chest, the only way to repair it is through surgery. Problem is, your counts again dipped down today, so surgery is not a good option right now for you, and quite frankly, this isn't a life threatening issue. So they repaired the line and will know tomorrow if it held. Regardless, next week, when your counts stabilize, you will again need surgery to install a new line. In the meantime, they needed to put an IV in your head to administer medicine. It's so hard to see that happen to you again and it reminds us way too much of our first week here with you when you had to have an IV in that same location. We'd forgotten what that was like and all the associated feelings that the memories of the first week brought with it. Those were very bad times, my friend, and we don't ever want to go back there again. Then to top it all off, your counts didn't rise like we expected, but fell instead. It's really one of those things that you can't predict, but still we try, and so far, we've been unsuccessful at guessing where things are headed from day to day. I really thought you were headed upward yesterday. Guess I was wrong...

Finally, we had to move rooms today to a different wing. We'd actually gotten really used to C714 and had made it a home away from home, if that's possible. So to move to a new room felt so foreign. By the time I had gotten back from work, your mom had the room all decorated again, but to me, it just didn't feel the same. I guess the good news is that we may only be in this room for a couple more weeks before we will get to leave for a little while. Your doctor told us today that a fourth round of ocean waves is on the horizon for next week. Once you get that round, we'll be able to leave the hospital for a little while. She's changing things up a little this time to try to go after the tumors that remain in your leg a little more than in the past. While this round won't include the desert sunset, she does think it might hit you a little harder overall, so we may be back in the hospital sooner than we would like. Nevertheless, as I have said before, we don't care what it will take, if it means leading you to recovery, we'll do whatever is asked of us...and you.

So much happened today, after many days of stability, that it really hit your mom hard. I know she had a difficult day dealing with everything that was going on. Days like this just really slap you in the face and remind you of the reality that has become your life. You may think you have things under control, but that couldn't be further from the truth. We're just passengers on this roller coaster sitting right beside you. And I can tell you from experience, my little friend, your mom is NOT a fan of scary rides. So do me a favor, give her a little break tomorrow and remind her that the stable and good days can easily make you forget about the difficult ones.

Be brave
Be strong
We love you!

WEDNESDAY, NOVEMBER 26, 2008

Brave Will,

This darn chemo has really taken a toll on you this time around. No matter how many days pass, it seems like your counts just cannot climb. Over the past five days you've been up one day and down the next. The doctors said it's likely that the marrow in your bones that helps to make those counts climb is just very tired right now. You've gotten such a high dose of chemo for three straight months with little time for a break, your body is just worn down. As a result, it's taking a lot longer for you to recover from the ocean waves. This leaves you still very sleepy and very nauseous when you try to eat. Sadly, those smiles are still few and far between. Your mom and I know you will eventually recover, we just can't help but be very impatient.

We did get you off of the morphine today so we were able to remove that line from your head once again. The line in your chest was repaired temporarily so they can at least feed medicine to you that way. It sounds like you'll need to go back into surgery next Thursday to install a new permanent line. You're a grizzled veteran at this surgery thing by now, so we're confident you'll do fine as always.

Because you still feel so yucky right now, your time with the family on Thanksgiving will be limited. We will be able to bring you to our big feast for just a short while. Fortunately, you'll be able to see lots of your relatives as we are expecting a gathering of over 30 family and friends in the banquet room at the hotel. We're just so thankful that we can all be together and that you'll be there with all of us. Even though we won't be able to have you there for too long, I'm certain your presence will raise everyone's spirits on this holiday. Thanksgiving is the perfect holiday for how all of us feel right now. We have so much to be thankful for and topping the list is the fact that you are still here enriching our lives. I'm sure I'll have much more to say when I write to you tomorrow, so tonight, I'll simply say "thank you"...

Be brave
Be strong
We love you!

THURSDAY, NOVEMBER 27, 2008

Brave Will,

Thankful that you got to spend your first Thanksgiving with 39 family and friends who all knew we needed to be with them on this special day

Thankful that you are still with us despite everything that you have gone through

Thankful for the doctors and nurses whose wisdom has allowed them to do everything in their power to make you healthy

Thankful that your story has been viewed over 107,000 times and has reached the entire world

Thankful that over 3,800 people have provided us with words of encouragement

Thankful that your life has been able to touch so many people and that you are helping other people in their own lives

Thankful for the ocean waves: Desert Sunset, Ocean Water, Yellow Flower, HaiChao, and Autumn Harvest

Thankful for the countless people who have provided us with more than we would have ever thought we needed (donations, rooms, food, presents for the boys, gift cards, etc.), but in the end truly do need

Thankful that a plan for your full recovery exists and that we are taking every step possible to get you there

Thankful that cancer may have knocked us down but has not buried our strength, perseverance, or unending love

Thankful that emotions like anger, resignation, despair, sadness, and grief may come, but they always go

Thankful that miracles can happen

Thankful that prayers, thoughts, and wishes can make a difference

Thankful for friendships that produce bonds strong enough to handle life's greatest challenges

Thankful that the support of family is enough to conquer mountains

Thankful for the two little boys who love their little brother and have made so many sacrifices to help you get better

Thankful to have your Mom in my life to get me through our darkest times

Thankful that you have entered our lives and have forever changed how we will live it

Happy 1st Thanksgiving, Will...

Be brave
Be strong
We love you!

SATURDAY, NOVEMBER 29, 2008

Brave Will,

I'm still trying to fully understand the events of yesterday. I decided to get a good night's sleep before I wrote to you so that things would be a little clearer in my mind. I'm not sure it did the trick. I can't say that things are worse after yesterday and I can't say that things are better. As your mom said, after everything we went through throughout the day on Friday, we really went in one big circle and are right back where we started Friday morning. But that's better than it could have been...

You see Will, since last week, there's been a few little things that are happening to you that were causing concern. Besides the normal chemo recovery stuff, you've been very nauseous (which should have passed by now), your temperatures have been lower than normal, you've been sleepier than normal, and you've just not looked yourself. They've been running a number of tests over the past few days and have been unable to find anything conclusive. Yesterday, they decided to give you an MRI on your brain to make sure nothing had come back that would most certainly cause some of the things they have been seeing.

Those MRIs are and will always be a stressful time for your mom and me. We let you go for an hour or two and are totally at the mercy of whatever the results end up being. It's a very helpless feeling. We've learned to expect the worse and hope for the best. When the doctor first came in with the results, we heard what we feared the most. Then about an hour later, the news we got from the same doctor was far different--a different interpretation, a different reading, a different analysis...we're not quite sure. But we do know the outcome changed drastically a few times over the course of two hours. Your mom and I felt like it was September all over again for a little while and then were relieved to hear that things weren't as bad as they originally seemed. If I'm being a little vague, it's because things are a little vague to us right now. We think things are no different than they were after your last MRI, which is good, great, miraculous, but we're not sure if something was seen to cause the concern they initially had. Confused, little buddy, just confused...

So they're still searching for answers about what's causing these symptoms. And I'm sure more tests will continue. I can't really tell you where things are headed until we get a chance to talk to your doctor on Monday.

We know we experienced one of the most frightening fire drills of our lives and that's enough to snap us back into reality, if that was needed at all. We know that these tests will make us question our strength and ability to cope should those days ever come. But lastly, we know we will continue to be thankful for each and every day that you are here with us.

Be brave
Be strong
We love you!

SUNDAY, NOVEMBER 30, 2008

Brave Will,

So each day over the past week, your mom and I have been trying to guess what your white blood counts are going to be each morning. Those are those ever important "counts" I keep telling you about. So day after day, I would guess they would go up, and would be disappointed that they actually fell lower. The doctors like to see that number higher than 6. Well, on Friday they finally climbed to 1.7 (after being between .1 and .5 all week). Yesterday, I guessed it would rise from 1.7 to 3.2 and they were only at 2.4. So today, I decided to be conservative and said they would be 3.7. Imagine my surprise when we found out they had climbed to 11.4! Wow--let the good times role. It's so easy to tell when your counts have risen--the smiles roll back in, you start singing like a little bird, and eat anything in site. You spend more time awake and actually seem to enjoy your exercise time. It's such a site to behold. It's sad that every day can't be like that, which every other 4-month old baby gets to experience. However, as we know well by now, you just aren't like every other 4-month old. So we learn to cherish those really good days. Usually when those good days come, it also means that the doctors are licking their chops to get their hands on you to begin the next round of ocean waves, and I am certain that will happen again this week. But in the meantime, we are going to take advantage of our opportunity to have our "normal" baby back again-- the one that is happy, smiling, and that you would never guess was sick.

So today, after spending the morning with Ben and Max, we spent the afternoon with just you in our hotel room. We all got to nap together, and then we gave you a feast. You were, of course, thrilled to see that football was on. It really is becoming a sight to behold to watch how you will crane and contort your neck in any way possible so that you can catch a glimpse of the game. You truly are your daddy's son...

In my last letter, I told you about our rough day we had on Friday. Tomorrow, I'm going to stick around the hospital in the morning to get a chance to speak to your primary doctor about everything we heard last week about your MRI. While we are definitely breathing a little easier now, we want to really fully comprehend what was seen, what wasn't seen, and what this means for you this week and beyond. I'm not sure that after Friday, your mom or I will ever feel safe again even if and when that day comes when you switch from being labeled a "cancer patient" to "cancer survivor". We realized how quickly that bad news can come, and while we've grown to not be surprised if that news does get delivered, we just don't know how we can ever prepare ourselves. So when your doctor enters our room tomorrow, we'll both take some really deep breaths, brace ourselves, and listen closely to where the road heads next...

Be brave
Be strong
We love you!

MONDAY, DECEMBER 01, 2008

Brave Will,

I can't believe it's December 1st. Normally, I would probably say something like, "I'm amazed at how quickly time has flown by." In this case, buddy, it feels like we've been going through this for three years, not three months. So the rise of a new month doesn't carry the same impact as you would expect.

Today started with a one-hour visit with your primary doctor. It's the thing I love about your doctor--she never makes us feel like she has any other place to be but in your room. I'm sure, after a long holiday weekend, and the start of a busy work week, she had plenty of work waiting for her on her desk. However, there she sat answering question after question from your mom and me. We certainly had a lot to ask her after everything that happened on Friday. One thing I have learned however, if you ask a doctor an hour's worth of questions, be prepared to get a day's worth of answers. My head was filled with so much information that I'm still trying to absorb everything she told us. So what did we learn this morning?

○ She is pretty certain that the initial MRI reading that was given to us on Friday wasn't accurate. The corrected reading that was later shared that day with us seems to be where things are currently at, which is to say, things haven't changed much, if at all, since your last MRI. Truly the biggest sigh of relief

○ So what was seen on Friday to cause the concern? Could have been a lot of things--dead cells, scar tissue, "artifacts", maybe even a small spot of cancerous cells. But certainly not anywhere near what was believed to be there and not anything to be threatened by...right now.

o With those concerns aside, we now begin to focus on Round 4 of the ocean waves. Things are going to change this time around. You'll get a break from the desert sunset this round (and likely next round as well). Instead, a different medicine will be substituted that may be better suited at attacking the tumor in your leg, while at the same time still maintaining things in your brain. The break from the desert sunset is needed to give your brain a break from the heavy, heavy stuff that can have some pretty substantial lingering effects. We'll need to come back to that eventually, but there's only so much of that you can get in a short amount of time.

o After round four, we will likely be discharged temporarily from the hospital to our "home" across the street. This will allow us all to be together day and night for at least a few days before you get readmitted for the next round.

o On Thursday, you'll have surgery to replace the central line that broke last week. In addition, you'll have some bone marrow removed to see if there is any evidence of cancer in your bones.

o On Friday, round four will start. Ideally, if you are able to bounce back quickly enough, you'll also get round five this month before Christmas. It will be close in terms of days to accomplish this, especially if you have a difficult recovery like the last round. It's really hard to imagine having to watch you endure two rounds in such a short amount of time.

o Some long term plans for the New Year--visiting a different hospital to talk about stem cell rescue; visiting a different hospital to talk about what to do with your leg (is surgery an option yet?); a biopsy of your left femur to see if the spot that shows on the scans is still active cancer cells or if they have died off. These little field trips will certainly dictate a lot of what we can and can't do in the future.

You see what I mean, Will? So much information in such a short amount of time. It helps me to write to you to sort it all out in my mind even though I'm certain at this point, you are wondering if you really need to know all of this medical mumbo jumbo.

Most importantly, today's conversation and Friday's events are such a constant reminder of how much of a struggle this will continue to be. We know that at any one of those meetings with your doctor, we could hear the word "reoccurrence"--it's just the nature of this type of cancer...it just keeps finding a way to come back. I keep hoping and praying that you will be different, but the statistics and studies say otherwise. We simply have to continue to believe that you will be the anomaly and you will be the miracle. In the meantime, we'll just continue to enjoy the fact that you are here with us and try not to get too caught up in the "what could happen" and "what might be"s. If you think of an easy way to do this, my little friend, please don't hesitate to share it with your mom and me...

Be brave
Be strong
We love you!

WEDNESDAY, DECEMBER 03, 2008

Brave Will,

Tomorrow, you'll have the fourth surgery of your short little life. You know you've been involved too many times with surgery when you begin to request certain anesthesiologists. I have to admit, I'm certainly less nervous this time around. The dangers and warnings they give don't really seem to apply to you. The procedure is relatively routine--they will replace the broken line that is inserted in your chest with a new one so that they can more easily administer medicines to you. It's fairly non-invasive and will hopefully allow you to have a quick recovery. While you are asleep, the doctors are also going to take a little snippet of bone marrow from your hip as well as some fluid from your spine so they can test those areas as well. All of these are done so that they can rule out the spread of your cancer to other parts of your body.

You are certainly ready for surgery--your counts have held above normal and your spirits are good. Smiles have been aplenty and your appetite is returning, especially with the newest addition of fruit to your diet. It's really bittersweet. We love seeing you smile, sing, eat, and coo, but know that it won't last for too much longer. On Friday, they'll start the next round of the ocean waves, and within a short time, you'll return to feeling pretty lousy. We just don't get to see you feeling good for that long, and when we do, then we know it's a sign that it's time to start the next round. As I have said before, as difficult as this is, we keep in perspective the reason we are here.

Once the next round ends, we can look forward to being discharged sometime next week. We'll take up residence across the street in the hotel for a few weeks to see how you are responding to the chemotherapy. Your mom is getting a crash course this week in nursing. She's learning how to flush your lines and administer your TPN. She's certainly been witness to a lot of nursing over the past three months, so I think she'll make an excellent caretaker for you. I'm going to learn a thing or two tomorrow so I can lend a hand as well. The sooner we learn these care tips, the sooner our next "new normal" can begin, no matter where our "home" is.

Be strong tomorrow, my little man, and let's move on to the next set of business.

Be brave
Be strong
We love you!

THURSDAY, DECEMBER 04, 2008

Brave Will,

All good. Today, was all good. Granted, we got into surgery about five hours later than we thought and the procedure took a little longer than was planned and we couldn't feed you for over twelve hours. But in the end, it was all good. You have been outfitted with a brand spanking new Hickman line. It's a different style and it now appears as though you have a garden hose coming out of you because the line is a bit larger than the one they removed today. It should help to have this bigger line in the future for procedures that might be needed, like stem cell harvesting. The doctor was also able to take a little snippet of bone from your hip to study the bone marrow. She also took out a little spinal fluid to test that as well. While she was there, she also gave you a little squirt of chemotherapy in your spinal area. All in all, you had a pretty eventful day.

Things are set to begin the next round of the ocean waves tomorrow. We're following a different treatment plan this time around and we learned a little more about it from your doctor. This treatment plan, while still doing a little work in your brain, will hopefully start to better attack your leg. Most of the medicines are the same but desert sunset will take a brief hiatus. It's going to be replaced by a new medicine (name coming soon). This plan will only last a couple of days and then if all goes well, we'll be discharged on Monday. Can you believe it? Now granted, it will likely be only for a few days, but still, all five of us will be able to be together for the entire day and night--no shifts, no babysitters, no split parenting; just a family of five under one roof (or in our case, all under the fourth floor). That's definitely something to look forward to...we can't wait.

Be brave
Be strong
We love you!

SATURDAY, DECEMBER 06, 2008

Brave Will,

Today was one of those days that really tested us. Your brother Ben was feeling sick off and on all day and even threw up a couple of times. In the meantime, you have definitely not been yourself. As a result, your mom, grandma, and I spent the day pinballing between the hotel room and hospital room trying to be everything to everyone, but really feeling inadequate in our skills to make our little boys feel better.

In Ben's case, I'm sure a good night's sleep will help him feel better. In your case, however, we're just not sure how to help...we never are. You were definitely a little uncomfortable yesterday but it intensified greatly today. At one point, earlier this evening, you were literally screaming in pain for roughly 30 minutes. It wasn't until the nurse gave you morphine that you finally settled down. It was great that the pain went away, but it didn't help us figure out why you were in pain in the first place. I am so incredibly frustrated that I can't help ease your pain in times like this. It seems like my only defense is to hold you close to me to ease your pain, and when that doesn't work, I'm out of options. Unfortunately, you can't tell us where it hurts and because there is so much to consider with your condition, it's very difficult to pinpoint what is causing the discomfort--is it typical baby stuff or pain from the chemotherapy or pain from the cancer or pain from the surgery Thursday or the new chest tube or a combination of all of these? You can really feel defenseless as a parent when your baby is screaming in agony and there is literally nothing you can do to ease the pain. It's just a hopeless feeling...I'm so sorry I couldn't help you tonight, my little man.

So a few new tests were run today to try to determine what is going on. One thing we do know--something is wrong and it's not just your mom and I noticing it. You just aren't the laid-back Will that the nurses have grown to know and love. When you act out of character, they definitely notice too. It sounds like they are going to keep looking for clues throughout the night and I am hoping something is found soon so they can give you some relief.

We did have a delay in starting this round of Ocean Waves. Instead of starting yesterday, your surgery ended up taking a little more out of you than we would have liked. As a result, they waited until today to start. You did receive a new medicine, a red one that we are calling Holiday Cheer. This round will be much quicker, in terms of delivery. They'll give you some more tomorrow, spend the next day flushing it out of your system and then it will be done. At that point, we could be in a position to be discharged. But again, with these other things going on, I'm not looking that far ahead or going in to next week with any set expectations. My only focus is on figuring out what hurts in your body and why.

I only hope that I can sleep tonight, put today behind me, and that when I awake tomorrow, this newest pain will be a distant memory.

Be brave
Be strong
We love you!

SUNDAY, DECEMBER 07, 2008
(Letter from Mom)

Hello my sweet baby boy,

As I begin writing to you my eyes are already filling with tears. It has nothing to do with last night, you slept fine. You were not quite yourself today and we continue to search for answers as to where this new pain is coming from, yet that is not why I am tearing up either. Today, buddy, I am crying tears of joy for all the amazing people that are in our lives. Some have been with us forever, and some are new friends.

Three months ago I would have never thought that I could say I was lucky considering I have a baby with cancer, yet buddy, we are. Today, a wonderful friend of our family put together a fundraiser at her salon. Not only did she, her husband and daughter arrange an amazing day, many others made it happen as well. I was speechless and overwhelmed to see all of these people come together for our family. Events like these, friends bringing dinner, a kind word, phone call, nurses and doctors who make us feel like family here, help Mommy and Daddy find the strength to make it to the next day. Years from now, I look forward to seeing you and your brothers volunteering to help another family make it to another day, like so many have done for us. As your daddy said today, if support and love could cure cancer, you would have checked out of the hospital weeks ago.

One of the women that came for a hair cut today inspired me and made me realize just how lucky we are. You see buddy, she lost her son Nick in October. She began her long road in July. In four short months, her beloved son was no longer with them. I am in awe of the fact that she came today to support our family while grieving for her own. She knows the road we are on--the exhaustion, fear, unknown-- and she would gladly keep doing it to have one more day. That is how we feel...we can do this forever baby, as long as you are with us.

So, we still have to figure out why you feel uncomfortable aside from the chemo, get your body healed from surgery, figure out where we go after these last drops of ocean waves flow through you, and so many other things. Yet for today buddy, we ARE the lucky ones...

Be brave
Be strong
We love you!

MONDAY, DECEMBER 08, 2008

Brave Will,

Your mom was nice to give me a break last night. It's important that you read her voice from time to time and she certainly has a wonderful way of showing you how much she cares (as if she really needs to do more). She has an amazing way with words, far more than she gives herself credit for. But we really did have an amazing day yesterday. Days like those have so much power that they give us enough strength to get through the potentially rough days to come. And just when we feel worked over again and don't know how we'll get through the next "thing", there's something else waiting for us to boost our spirits and spur us on.

The fourth round of the Ocean Waves has come and gone. This was a different mix this time around and the addition of Holiday Cheer is sure to not make you very cheerful in the days to come. Even though the Desert Sunset was removed this time, the reality is that this concoction might actually hit you harder than the previous cycles. In fact, you are already starting to show some signs of wear and tear from this most recent round. As a result, our plans to leave for a few days have been foiled again. A wise man once sang, "You can check out any time you like, but you can never leave." It seems like our only chances to leave these days appear to be the brief 3-5 hour "jailbreaks". The doctors just feel like things are already going south. In all likelihood, if we were to leave tomorrow, it would be a matter of days, if not hours, before we would have to be readmitted. I was admittedly excited at the thought of having us all together as much as I try not to think too far ahead. The boys were busy decorating the tree in preparation of your arrival, but they understand that it's important that you stay right where you are so the doctors can keep a close eye on you.

So you'll be in the hospital for at least two more weeks. That puts us right at the two month mark that they told us to expect back in October. But this at least gives us hope that we could get you "home" for Christmas. Obviously, this will depend entirely on how well you recover from this round of treatment, and judging by the early signs, this is going to be a tough go for you.

Nevertheless, we're keeping our spirits up during this holiday season. Without question, this will be unlike any Christmas season that any of us have experienced before. But all things considered, the memories that we build during this month will likely place very high on our all-time list of Christmas memories. There's no doubt about it, our Christmas miracle has arrived a little early.

Be brave
Be strong
We love you!

TUESDAY, DECEMBER 09, 2008

Brave Will,

When I opened the door to the hotel room tonight, the best present ever was waiting for me under the tree. Fortunately, I didn't have to wait 16 days to open it. That's right buddy, you gave me an early present. It seems the doctors had a change of heart this morning and decided to discharge you after all. So when I walked in, you were there, no strings attached. Our family was all finally together. It was quite an overwhelming feeling at first, and I'm still letting it sink in that when I go to bed tonight, all of us will be sleeping in the same room for the first time since September 11th. It's been almost three months since your mom stole the covers from me in the middle of the night and I can't wait for it to happen again tonight.

I'm thrilled, excited, happy, overjoyed, and I'll let you in on a little secret about one more emotion...I'm scared out of my mind. As I looked around the room and saw the medicines, syringes, flushes, tubes, and machines, I began to realize that all of those things are still with you too. Just because we left the hospital behind doesn't mean we've left the cancer behind too (as much as we'd all like to). The reality of the situation just sat there scattered around the room staring me back in the face. This is what life is like now, what life is like outside the safety net of the hospital, doctors, and nurses.

Your mom has been getting crash courses in taking care of your needs every single day and night. The nurse spent two hours with her in the room tonight showing everything that she needs to do from sunrise to sunset. I sat there amazed at your mom's knowledge and poise as she plunged, connected, and administered all that "stuff". At least I know you are in the best hands possible. I wonder if I'll be able to possess that same confidence when it comes time for me to take care of you--it scares me to think that we are in control of this process now.

For now, I think I'll let your mom become the expert of the family. When she is ready, I'll gladly become her student and learn everything there is to give you the best possible care you require while we have you at home. You could be here for a day, a week, or maybe even until after Christmas, so we want to do everything in our power to keep you healthy and happy while you enjoy your stay at Hotel Hladun.

Welcome home...

Be brave
Be strong
We love you!

FRIDAY, DECEMBER 12, 2008

Brave Will,

Well, it was fun while it lasted...

Today, a series of things led to you being re-admitted into the hospital. It was not entirely unexpected and your doctor told us last weekend that even if you did get discharged, there would be a good chance that you would be back in the hospital fairly quickly. Still, we were hoping you would be able to fight off all those nasty things that can get you when you're feeling down and out. But it wasn't meant to be. We kind of knew last night that things were starting to head downhill. You had been throwing up all day and barely got any sleep last night. You got a small fever in the middle of the night that went away just as quickly as it came, and you looked very pale. All signs that you were probably going to need extra attention today. Sure enough, when you had your regular appointment at the clinic this morning, you had a pretty high fever and were immediately admitted.

It was disappointing to say the least, but we'll rebound quickly. It's uncertain how long your next stay will be. You may just need to stay there until the fever breaks, or they may want to keep you until your counts come back up (and we know how long that can take). Regardless, we're still keeping our fingers crossed that you'll be let out by Christmas. Your counts have bottomed out, so we've got a fair amount of time to wait for you to start feeling good again.

Admittedly, it was difficult having everything be back to "normal" over the past three days and trying to get adjusted to all living in a hotel room. I definitely struggled with being a dad to all three of my boys, but I wouldn't trade the time we all got to spend together. Your mom was right when she said we need to maximize every opportunity we have when all of us can be together. In my haste to try to get things back to the way they were, which is nearly impossible right now, I lost sight of that. So I'm glad she made sure we did those little things to make sure we didn't forget this brief time in our life. I guess the hard part, I quickly realized, is that when you do get to come home, it will be impossible to go back to the way things were. I really want that to happen, but it just can't...too much has happened to allow that to happen.

So, we're back to our reality; you're mom is staying at the hospital with you and I'm with Ben and Max at the hotel. We had a nice day today because of the snow day and didn't have to go anywhere. We were able to take your brothers with you to the clinic and they got to go "shopping" there to pick out gifts for you (and themselves) for Christmas. But at 6:30, your mom headed back to the hospital to see you and I put the boys to bed, a ritual we've grown very accustomed to. Today was three months since we first were admitted into this fate, and while earlier this week it felt like we were beginning to make some progress, today showed us that there's still a long, long way to go no matter how long the last three months have really felt...

Be brave
Be strong
We love you!

SATURDAY, DECEMBER 13, 2008

Brave Will,

It was a hard day for you today as the worst of the effects of the ocean waves have begun to take their toll. It appears as though you've definitely hit bottom once again and it will probably be a few days before you start to rebound. So, the key to keeping you happy is to try and give you plenty of rest and find the right combination to make you relatively pain-free. That means it's back to the pain medication, which we've come to accept as a needed part of the recovery process. We know it won't last forever and will certainly allow you to feel more comfortable, which is the key to giving you the rest you need.

You were able to spend almost the entire day with Grandma as your mom and I were with Ben and Max all day long. We took them to the dentist this morning and met some wonderful people there who are being so helpful to our family. I hope someday to be able to take you there to meet them as well. Your brothers were very brave and helpful as the dentist checked their teeth. It made us wonder--when will you start to cut your own teeth? And when that happens, will we know the difference between that pain and the other random pain you experience throughout the month? It's just one of the tricky things that we'll need to be aware of that normally we would have never even thought much of.

After the dentist, we took your brothers to the new house to see how that was coming along--it's getting closer, and we're really starting to get excited about moving in to the new place. We figure we're about 4-6 weeks away from calling it "home" for good.

All in all, it was a great day to be with your brothers. If we can't all be together as one family, being able to spend quality time with them is so important to your mom and me. We need them to know that our lives, despite all that we're going through, can't revolve solely around what's happening to you. Those little snippets of time where we can do silly things like sing songs in the car, wrestle on the bed, and watch Christmas specials together are so meaningful to them, and even more so to your mom and dad.

This juggling act will likely have to continue for at least another week or so before we have another shot to all be together again. Obviously, there will be a lot more times in the future when we're going to have to figure out how to be in two separate places at the same time. But I know that your mom and I are starting to get a good handle on the needs of not only you, but of your two older brothers so that we can continue to provide all that is possible to be everything to everyone in our little family.

Be brave
Be strong
We love you!

MONDAY, DECEMBER 15, 2008

Brave Will,

Not much new to report, but since I didn't get a chance to write last night to you, I wanted to make sure I had a chance to say "happy 5 month birthday"! Are you sure you aren't eight months old yet? It really feels like you have been with us for so much longer than the calendar indicates. You certainly are an old weathered soul by now who's experienced so much more than any 5-month-old out there. I can picture you sitting around when you are 5-years-old telling your friends, "And this scar is from a brain surgery...and this scar is from my first line that they had to insert into my chest...and this scar..."

So your days recently have pretty much revolved around you sleeping the days away. You're not a happy camper when you're awake, so it's just as well that you spend your days and nights sleeping. Also, with the amount of morphine going through you right now to help you deal with those nasty mouth sores, I suspect that when you are awake, you must be in a pretty "interesting" place. Even when your eyes are open, you seem to be off in a distant place--La La Land, we like to call it. But at least in that place, I'm sure there are lots of happy sights and sounds, and pain is nowhere to be found. We'll let you enjoy that special place for a few more days until your counts start to rise and those sores clear up. Then, we'll gladly take you back into reality and replace the drugs with hugs...

Be brave
Be strong
We love you!

WEDNESDAY, DECEMBER 17, 2008

Brave Will,

Things are still pretty much the same as they have been all week. Your counts are still dreadfully low and you're receiving platelet and blood transfusions every other day to help you recover. However, those little signs that we look for are starting to appear. You smiled for your grandma today and she said she almost got a laugh out of you. Tonight, when the boys and I came to visit you, I was able to coax a few small smiles out of you as well. That's a great sign that you're starting to turn the corner. I would expect that over the next couple of days, you'll start taking the pacifier again, then back to your bottle and then finally eating again. During that time, we should also be able to take you off of the morphine and get you back into reality a little more. As of right now, we're still hopeful that we'll get you back "home" in the hotel by early next week, with time to spare before Christmas. What makes this even better than your last visit home was that last week, you were on the verge of crashing so you're time home was difficult on you. Next week, you'll be peaking into tip-top shape so we'll get you on your best days. I'm expecting lots of smiling and talking all week!

The plan (at least as of today) is to have you home all next week through Christmas and the following weekend. Our doctor is trying to schedule a trip for us down to NYU during the week before New Year's to meet with a doctor to talk about stem cells. I've mentioned this to you before, but haven't really shared what it all means. Basically, in January, they are going to take some of your stem cells out of your body and store them. These cells will help down the road when you start to have more problems recovering from all of these heavy doses of Ocean Waves. Think of it as a bank that you can use to withdraw healthy cells to make you feel better again after all the chemotherapy. I'm sure I'll learn a lot more about how it all works when we meet with the doctor in New York City, so I'll give you more details as soon as I have a better handle on this.

But hey, that's still a few weeks off, and if there's one thing we've all learned through this, it's that we should never look too far ahead in the future. Our focus is solely on getting your counts back up to normal and to get you out of the hospital in time to spend your first Christmas with your two older brothers who can't wait to tell you all about Santa Claus and the joy that December 25th brings...

Be brave
Be strong
We love you!

FRIDAY, DECEMBER 19, 2008

Brave Will,

Home for the holidays...

I'm looking across the hotel room at you sleeping soundly in your crib. You've made it home again, little buddy, and hopefully, this time it will be for a lot longer. Your counts, while still needing to rise, are high enough that the doctor felt comfortable sending you "home" with mom today. The plan is to keep you safe and sound with us through the holidays for at least a week. A whole week with all of us together...the perfect Christmas gift.

So tonight is just your typical, "snowed in on a Friday night with your entire family in a hotel room across the street from the hospital" that I'm sure many have experienced :) Your mom is excited to spend the night with Ben and Max, something she hasn't been able to do for more than one night at a time. Likewise, it will be nice for me to be able to see you for more than 30 minutes a day over the next week. We're going to be busy little man, but I'm sure you'll be ready for a little activity at this point in your life.

Looking forward to the days to come...

Be brave
Be strong
We love you!

MONDAY, DECEMBER 22, 2008

Brave Will,

We've been enjoying life as a family of five so much, I've been neglecting my duties of writing to you. It's not that I haven't thought about it, it's just that life has been strolling along so merrily, it's almost like these letters don't need to exist while our life imitates "normalcy". So this weekend, we got to take you out for the day on Saturday. On Sunday, we were pretty much snowed in all day at the hotel, which was just about the best thing that could have happened. All five of us got to spend the day together "doing nothing". You lounged on the couch with your brother Max, watched your brothers make Christmas cookies, got to take your first "real" bath in months, and just hung with the guys. Your mood has been spectacular--lots of smiles, activity, and eating. We knew there was a five-month-old baby in there somewhere. It's nice to see it come out once in a while.

We're going to have you in this tip-top shape for another week, which is all we could hope for. We're going to enjoy Christmas with our families on Wednesday and Thursday. On Monday, we'll head down to NYU in New York City to meet with a doctor about your stem cells and how we might be able to use them in the future. This should give us a short-term plan for the next few months. Then, to bring in the New Year, you'll start round 5 on New Year's Eve. Not sure exactly what will be included in the cocktail this time around, but we're sure to have some of our chemo favorites on the playlist.

Your mom and I had some blood work done about two weeks ago and sent it off along with yours to a doctor that specializes in the genetic makeup of brain tumors, including the one you have. The results of your test that we got back today weren't entirely surprising given your diagnosis. You have what they call a germline mutation in the genes that make up all the cells in your body. Because your tumors are in multiple locations, the diagnosis was expected. What this means is that your body has a predisposition to grow tumors because the mutation takes place in a part of your body that helps to fight off danger as cells develop. Not really what we wanted to hear, but it certainly didn't surprise us. We're very clear, as we have always been, that you're in for a fight, and it won't be easy. Nevertheless, you shown so much progress in three months, I can't even view the day's news as a setback, just a another reality that we'll all deal with.

But for now, let's just enjoy the holidays, enjoy health, and enjoy having you with us as Christmas rapidly approaches.

Be brave
Be strong
We love you!

WEDNESDAY, DECEMBER 24, 2008

Brave Will,

Merry 1st Christmas!

I still remember the morning of the day we found out what kind of cancer you had. Your doctor didn't know the exact diagnosis yet, but she hinted that it was not going to be good news later that day. I can vividly recall her telling us that one of the nurses had asked her if she would be able to get you to your first Christmas. I'll never forget what that felt like hearing those words. Three months ago, that was...only three months, and there was a strong feeling that you wouldn't be here with us on this night. Looking back at just how short that was, three months was just not long enough to have you with us.

So as we sit at the doorstep of Christmas day, I now know you're going to be here with us tomorrow. I was too superstitious to even relay this story to you before tonight. But I feel safe in telling you now. You hit a big milestone and I'm sure there will be another one waiting for you after tomorrow.

I don't know if I feel lucky or not for having you with us. It should be a foregone conclusion that I should get to spend every one of my remaining Christmases on this earth with all three of my boys. But I am becoming all too well aware that this disease is keeping a number of families without a son or daughter on Christmas Day for the first time, and that continues to frustrate, discourage, and devastate me. You just can take nothing for granted in the fragile lives we lead. To think that I'm sitting in a hotel room on Christmas Eve would have been beyond comprehension 12 months ago. Now I know there is no where else I need to be. My perspective on life seems to change by the day, and I'm so keenly aware of the good fortunes that we have had to be where we are today. To know if those good fortunes will continue for weeks, months, or years would be strictly a guess and as much as I have asked Santa Claus to bring me a crystal ball, I'm not sure that wish will come true.

So tonight, I simply applaud the small milestones that you have achieved, respect the good fortunes that have been laid upon our family since you were stricken, and give all of my sincerest thoughts to those out there that have been so deeply impacted by this awful disease. They should never have to walk alone down this long and painful road.

Lastly, on your behalf, I want to thank everyone who has done so much to make this Christmas meaningful and memorable for our entire family. I don't think your mom and I could have mustered up the energy necessary to make Christmas as special as I know it will be for Ben and Max tomorrow. The devotion, kindness, and generosity of so many people in our lives will surely make this a Christmas we will never forget...

Be brave
Be strong
We love you!
Merry Christmas

MONDAY, DECEMBER 29, 2008

Brave Will,

We are just soaking up every minute of "Healthy Will" that we have been given. I'll admit, as much as I am proud and in awe of "Brave Will", I'm a much bigger fan of "Healthy Will". Still, you have been nothing short of the baby that every mom and dad dreams of over the last week. We have enjoyed having our little baby boy home with us again and feeling just fine. We've been able to get away from the hotel for a few days to enjoy time at your Nana and Poppie's house, where we were living before all of this started in September. It's given your mom a chance to spend time with her family and given me a chance to spend time at the new house doing some work. We're getting closer and closer to giving you a real home to come home to after your stays in the hospital.

Today, your mom and I took you to the Big Apple to meet with a doctor down there. We talked all about something called stem cells. These are the cells that your body uses to create all kinds of other cells. They can be very helpful in helping you recover from some of these heavier rounds of Ocean Waves that you have been getting. Believe it or not, and don't get mad at me, there are even heavier rounds that we may use in the future. If we choose to do this, this doctor will use those stem cells to help your body recover from the impact of the medicines that are used in those heavy-duty rounds. We'll need to meet with your doctor later this week to lay out a plan for next month. We'll need to head back to NYU at some point after your next round of treatment so they can take those stem cells out of your body and store them for you to use at a later time. I'm amazed at science every time I find out about one of these procedures. In this one, they take the blood out of you, shake it all up, remove just the helpful stem cells from the blood, and then put it right back into your body like it never left. Pretty crazy, huh?

So we get to enjoy our time with "Healthy Will" for another three days before the next round of Ocean Waves start. That means we'll get to bring in the New Year with you right by our side. If you're good, we'll let you stay up to watch the ball drop. But we want you to get some rest that night because the next day, you'll get readmitted to the hospital so they can start prepping your body for the chemotherapy that will start on Friday--Happy New Year! Hopefully, this round won't hit you as hard as the doctor is going to lower the amount of Holiday Cheer this time, which is what floored you in December. If all goes well, our stay could be brief and you could be discharged by next week.

Regardless, we've been able to have you with us for over a week now, and it is a time in our lives that we will never, ever forget. We know how important it is to take advantage of every moment that the five of us can be together, and I think we've been able to do that. You just can't predict how often or when these times will happen again, so we're thrilled to have these last two weeks to be a family again.

Be brave
Be strong
We love you

THURSDAY, JANUARY 01, 2009

Brave Will,

Happy New Year, my little friend...

Right on cue, you started to stir just a few minutes before midnight last night. Naturally, your mom and I took that as a sign that you wanted to join us to bring in the New Year, so we scooped you up out of the crib and shared hugs and kisses with you and your godparents.

Admittedly, I am more than ready to put 2008 behind me. While I know I was blessed during that year to have you enter our lives, I also felt a pain I never thought I would have to experience in my lifetime. The pain still exists but I'm ready to view this new year with renewed optimism. I'm ready to take the next steps toward something the medical profession calls NED (no evidence of disease). We've cleared some large hurdles to try to get there, but now is the time where we've got to make some major strides. The future is no clearer than it was three months ago, but the key thing is that we are all here three, nearly four months, later looking ahead to 2009. That accomplishment that continues to astound so many is one we will cherish for our lifetime.

I was listening to the radio the other day and they were interviewing a basketball coach and asked him about his New Year's resolutions. He responded to the question by saying that he had no resolutions, only his continued wish that his wife and children continue to be healthy. I thought, yup, that's all I want too. I never thought that much about it and it all seemed too simple to give it more than a moment's attention, but the health of my children is all that drives me at this point in my life. I figured it was one of those things that just happened--of course my sons would all live healthy lives--maybe a broken arm or scraped knee every now and again, but never anything that would stop me in my tracks. But here I sit, and your health and the health of Ben and Max is all I can focus on. How do I protect my sons from all that lurks? You think you have everything covered and have taken all the right precautions, but what I find is that as a dad, there is only so much I can do.

So what am I left with? Simply wishing, with whatever power and control I have left, that good health returns to our family. In 2009, my wishes for a happy year are simple: have the good fortune to be able to continue to fight this disease; do all we can to make sure you exit 2009 healthier than you started it; and of course, NED...

Be brave
Be strong
We love you!

SUNDAY, JANUARY 04, 2009

Brave Will,

It's been back to business as usual this weekend. On Friday, your mom brought you back over to the hospital to begin the next round of Ocean Waves. No question about it, it was infinitely more difficult this time around than the previous four. We had been able to spend two full weeks together as a family and you were acting as healthy as ever. But inevitably, we need to bring you back to that place that has conquered so much of our lives since September. Tonight, when I came to see you, I realized how quickly I forgotten what that walk felt like and the halls of the hospital weren't nearly as familiar as I expected them to be.

We're all feeling a little troubled right now with things. Last week we noticed that your right leg was looking a little larger than it had been. Of course, we were hoping it was just us being neurotic parents, but your doctor felt the same way when she saw you on Thursday. They did an MRI of your leg on Friday, and while it was a quick one and you were only sedated for it (which can alter the pictures they are able to take), the results did show some small growth. Not surprising to us, but certainly nothing we had hoped for. This immediately has changed the treatment planned for this round. The Holiday Cheer that they added last month was just as quickly removed from your plan--no point in giving you something that made you so sick and wasn't helping you at all. Instead your doctor is going back to the original plan with Yellow Flower, Ocean Water, HaiChao, and Desert Sunset. They're eliminating Autumn Harvest this time around because it's starting to affect the platelets in your blood. The issues are starting to pile up a little bit and we're all trying to get a handle on things before they go astray. You'll be getting these medicines until Tuesday and then hopefully, by weeks end, we'll be able to bust you out again for a little bit.

I guess what's most concerning to your mom and me, is what this all means for the future. When we saw tremendous progress in your brain and leg in October, there was a direct correlation--if one thing was going well, they all were. So clearly, we have that same fear going the other way now. They are going to do another MRI tomorrow where they will give you anesthesia. This will allow them to take the right pictures that they weren't able to do on Friday. I'm sure I have told you in the past that MRIs are the absolute worst for your mom and me. We wait hours for them to do the procedure and then just wait some more for someone to come and give the results, good or bad. Usually we find out that day--sometimes we have to wait until the next day. It's the perfect definition of helpless. But as you know, these pictures that are taken are critical and tell us so much about how things are going inside of your tiny little body. But still...ugh, I just hate the whole process.

We'll brace ourselves for whatever we learn tomorrow, and as always, pray for the best, prepare for the worst, and hope for something that falls in between. We've been down this road too many times to get caught off guard and we've even had "fire drills" to prepare us for what could be at any time. Regardless of what we find out from these scans, you've shown that you can handle anything that seems to be thrown your way, and I have no doubt that this will just be a small pothole in your journey...

Be brave

Be strong

We love you!

MONDAY, JANUARY 05, 2009

Brave Will,

Well, we're breathing a small sigh of relief tonight at the results of your MRI today. When the tumor in your leg shrunk this fall, the same thing was happening in your brain. Fortunately, the reverse has not been true. It appears as though the tumor in your leg has gotten a little larger. This needs to be confirmed with an official reading tomorrow, but you can see there has been a change over the past few weeks. However, the doctor said your "brain is beautiful" which was music to your mom's and my ears. The scan still shows no tumor growth in your brain and very little evidence of any mass at all. I really felt the thigh-brain correlation was going to work against us today, and am so grateful to hear otherwise. We've just bought ourselves a little more time, yet again.

Now for the bad stuff--they did do a hearing test while you were asleep today and found some loss in both of your ears. Again, this was something your mom and I suspected recently when we didn't see you reacting to some of the louder sounds that were going on around you. There is still hearing in both ears, but the ability to hear higher pitch sounds seems to have diminished. This is a result of the Yellow

Flower that you have received over the past months and is a common side effect--kind of a necessary evil that we were prepared for. They'll do some more tests tomorrow to get a better idea of the potential issues.

But the bigger battle is with the pesky disease that resides in your right leg. Unlike the brain, this mass seems to be fighting the chemo a lot more, which is a little surprising because we would have thought if the Ocean Waves washed away the tumor in one area it would be likely to do the same elsewhere, but that has not been the case. But we now have a new mission--finding a way to control that disease in your leg while trying to minimize long term impact. The options for your leg are certainly greater than they are for your brain, but the consequences are still nevertheless pretty severe. We're trying to do what's best for you little man, but there aren't a lot of great choices available to us. We'll now most likely need to meet with some orthopedic experts over the coming weeks to figure out the best way to attack this problem. Part of me can picture nothing but you running around with your brothers outside in five years, but I know the decisions we might have to make may prevent that from happening. However, making sure you are still with us six months, a year, or five years from now will win out against any future portrait I may have painted in my mind.

Each day--new challenges to face, new decisions to be made, and new victories to celebrate...

Be brave
Be strong
We love you!

THURSDAY, JANUARY 08, 2009

Brave Will,

Round Five of the Ocean Waves is in the books. It was administered pretty close to rounds 1-3 with the exception of Autumn Harvest being removed. You've already passed the Desert Sunset through you so you're in a good position to be discharged tomorrow. How long you get to stay home will depend entirely on your ability to avoid a fever. Last month, that only ended up being three days. However, that was a different kind of treatment that the doctor knew would put a hurtin' on you, and it did. This might be different because you have generally responded pretty well to this type of treatment. Time will tell, but we're happy to be able to get you home again to the hotel. We're hopeful that by your next round, when they discharge you, we'll be able to really take you home to your own house with your own room and your own crib. I can't wait to show you the new place. I just know you and your brothers are going to love it.

All told, you're holding up pretty well this week. You managed to continue to eat throughout the whole treatment, and you haven't stopped smiling yet. I know this is old hat to you by now, but still, you're showing a strength that continues to astound us. I imagine that in a couple of days, you'll finally hit the floor and need to spend most of your days sleeping, but for now, you've really kept your spirits up, and in doing so, have kept your mom and mine up as well.

Your mom is already working with you on some sign language this week. This is something she did with both Ben and Max to help them communicate things like "please", "thank you", "more", "mommy", and "daddy". It really helped them communicate to us earlier than they would have normally been able to say those words. In your case, we want to get you comfortable early on using those signs should we ever need to continue to use them. Besides, it's a great skill to learn (and I suspect, looks great on a college application!).

It's strange that just a short time ago, I was pretty nervous about them sending you home after getting chemotherapy. Now I'm hoping, hoping that you will fight off any fevers tonight so they can release you tomorrow. Everyone told us that this would happen eventually, but with your condition, I just felt so comfortable having you stay at the hospital month after month. Now I get what they were saying. That hospital is not going anywhere and will be there whenever we need it. But the time that we have together as a full family is so indefinite and so inconsistent, that we just have to take advantage of those days every month when we are giving the green light.

So if they give you the okay tomorrow, don't hesitate to pack your bags and head for the exits. I'll be waiting here for you with open arms...

Be brave
Be strong
We love you!

SATURDAY, JANUARY 10, 2009

Brave Will,

OK, I'll admit it. I was grumbling and complaining when I was walking back over to the hospital at 9:00 last night because you didn't end up getting discharged on Friday. I wasn't in the best of moods as a result, and it was probably a good thing that I didn't end up writing to you last night--it would have been a whole bag of negativity, and I had LOTS to say.

Fortunately, cooler heads, and extreme fatigue prevailed and I fell asleep instead. It was a long night, and even though you weren't sick like I've seen you in the past, you definitely weren't in the sleeping mood, so we had lots of "quality time" from 2:30 until around 6:00 this morning. Guess who's feeling fatigued again?

The main reason you had to stay was because your Desert Sunset level was a little higher than the doctors like, so they need to keep giving you the "rescue drug" which is not something your mom or I can give you here at the hotel. Also, there was some concern about your blood levels and possible rash, so they held on to you for another night.

So today, I left to spend another day working at the new house and took the boys to spend the day with their cousins. Your mom called me around noon to let me know that the doctor came in a said that you were likely going to be staying at least until Monday. If there's one thing you should know about your mom--she has an amazing gift of gab. She can talk and talk, whether it be arguing, pleading (that's how you came into our life), negotiating, or defending, that woman can talk her way into any situation. So needless to say, by the time she got done with the doctor, you were on your way to being discharged and spending at least a few days with the family. She'll bring you to clinic on Monday and they'll determine if we can continue to stay out. This will happen on Wednesday and Friday as well, so there are certainly no guarantees that this will be a long stay.

So tonight, your mom and I are sitting on the couch in the hotel staring at you sleeping next to us. It's nice to have you home again, little buddy...

Be brave
Be strong
We love you!

TUESDAY, JANUARY 13, 2009

Brave Will,

Not much new to share with you tonight but I felt the need to write to you. I've been amazed at how well you have been doing responding to this round of chemotherapy. You've still managed to avoid a return trip to the hospital which is a great sign and something we have yet to avoid in the previous four rounds. Also, while you've still gotten sick a lot, you don't seem to be struggling as much as we have seen in the past. And as always, our tell-tale sign, you've squeezed out a few smiles from time to time. Usually we don't see those until things start heading north, but we know we're still a week or so away from that. So all things considered, we're in a pretty good place right now.

I spent some time tonight talking to your doctor about your progress and what the next steps are. It's clear we have to address the disease that still exists in your leg as this is one area that appears to be active and potentially dangerous. I think I mentioned recently to you that the options for fighting the disease in this location are certainly greater than the options for fighting the disease in your brain. That being said, the options that exist are still not ones that your mom and I can easily comprehend. We've discussed this all before in the abstract, thinking we wouldn't have to make such choices, but it's clear that your doctor is ready for us to make a decision and move on it. She is having us meet next week with a doctor that specializes in cancers that appear in the leg. He will talk to us about our options and what he thinks is best. Your doctor has already expressed to us what she thinks is your best hope, so now your mom and I just need to come to terms with whatever we decide to do. What it boils down to is that few people thought you had a chance four months ago. But the progress you have shown has made everyone fall in love with you and because of that, no one wants to take any chance that could lose you. To get to that point, we may have to take some aggressive stances that would normally be avoided if we didn't think you could beat this thing. The hard part for your mom and I is that being aggressive with this still doesn't guarantee you the outcome that we all hope and pray for. What it does do is eliminate the possibility that the active disease in your leg will cause the cancer to spread to other areas of your body--it removes something else from the equation. The brain is seemingly under control right now; the area of skin on your back is easily removed; the tumor in your leg, however, is the tricky one and therefore has to be taken out of the equation one way or another. So your mom and I will do a lot of talking, research, and thinking between now and when we meet with the leg doctor. We'll ask him lots of questions and hopefully get the guidance we need to give you every chance possible to survive this thing.

Did you know that tomorrow is your 1/2 year birthday? Normally, a day like that might slide by, but not this year and not with this baby. The lens I choose to view life through right now is so magnified that those little things have such great magnitude. I'm not looking past any small milestone, minor accomplishment, or seemingly inconsequential achievement. Hitting six months, and doing as well as you are currently doing, is such an astounding feat, it has to be celebrated. I've often imagined your first birthday and how I fully expect it to be the biggest party on the planet. To know we are halfway there, when there were so many doubts we would get to this point, is something that should cause all of us to just pause, shake our heads and smile.

Be brave
Be strong
We love you!

FRIDAY, JANUARY 16, 2009

Brave Will,

Still holding strong, little man. Sure, your counts have dropped and you're still getting sick frequently, but your spirit and mood through the past week hasn't dipped. I was able to yank the most adorable little giggle out of you tonight--the first one that I've heard from you. Don't think for one minute that I'm not going to keep trying now to get more and more.

Your trip to the clinic today was long as you needed both blood and platelets. The Ocean Waves have definitely taken its toll on your platelets, and they just don't seem to bounce back. As a result, you've needed to get transfusions three times this week. There's no question we need to be careful with the amount of chemo you will get in the future because those platelets are getting harder and harder to grow in your body.

Your mom talked with the doctor today and she agreed with your mom that now would be a good time to make the clean break from the hotel. So on Sunday, we're going to finally check out and finally move back home to your Nana and Poppie's for the first time since September 12th. We're so relieved to be finally getting away. It was a blessing to be so close to the hospital for so long, especially when we felt far from comfortable being anything further than 3 minutes away from the hospital. But, like everything else, we're feeling better and better about establishing ourselves in our new home with our new normal, and this is the next logical step. We're probably about three weeks or so from being able to move into the new home and we're so excited to discover what life will look like when we're finally all together in our own home. Getting you through those doors seemed like a distant dream back in September, and now we're just weeks away.

So over the next few days as your counts remain low, we'll do everything in our power to keep you safe from fevers and sickness so that we'll only need one home, one place to sleep, one place to eat, and one place to live together as a family.

Be brave
Be strong
We love you!

TUESDAY, JANUARY 20, 2009

Brave Will,

Well, we're settling back in at your Nana and Poppie's house. I'm sure things are a little chaotic for them, but it's been so nice for your mom and me to have everyone together in one place. We're awfully lucky that they are both so welcoming and patient as we spend the next few weeks all under the same roof.

I gotta say, things are actually starting to feel routine right now, and I never thought I would feel that way. It's funny how life works though. When you were first diagnosed, I couldn't imagine life outside of the hospital--how would we be able to take care of you without the nurses right there by our side? Then once we got a taste of life outside the hospital, we couldn't wait to get more and more time away in the hotel--we were ready to handle things ourselves. At that point, we couldn't imagine living any further away from the hospital than the hotel. However, right after the New Year, we knew it was time--we were tired of the hotel life. We were ready to move on to the next phase, and just when that feeling hit, we were allowed to check out. It seems like in our life these changes don't happen until we are actually ready for what's next. And just when we think we can't take another day of our current situation, bang, we're ready to move on. It's funny how that all seems to just fall into place.

So life is good in our life up north from Albany Med. Your mom is still taking you to the hospital clinic every Monday, Wednesday, and Friday, but so far, you've only been a visitor and not become a resident once again. Your counts have started to climb once again, so we know you're getting ready for the next round of Ocean Waves. However, we may put that next round on hold for a little while longer.

Tomorrow, we're going to meet with a doctor to talk about what options we have in regards to treating your leg. We know there's not too many choices left for you in regards to treating your leg with just medicine. My secret wish over the past week was that your leg would miraculously shrink and there would be little need for a discussion. Unfortunately, no luck with that. So we'll see what tomorrow brings and be ready for the next turn in the road. Regardless of what we hear, discuss, and decide, we're never going to look past the fact that we are even in a position to be able to have these discussions and that you'll be sitting right there beside us ready for whatever challenge life presents you with next.

Be brave
Be strong
We love you!

WEDNESDAY, JANUARY 21, 2009

Brave Will,

Throughout this whole process, we've been faced with a lot of decisions that may appear to be, on the surface, difficult to make. However, when you dig a little deeper, you quickly realize there really wasn't much of a decision to make. When we met with the doctor today about your leg, I went into the meeting wondering if this would be one of those easy decisions or a difficult one? As I left the meeting, having made the decision with your mom, I'm not quite sure. On one hand, there is no question that what we decided to do today was by far the most difficult thing we have chosen to do to treat you. On the other hand, I'm not sure there was really another option available for you.

You see, little buddy, today we made the decision to have your right leg removed. Even as I type this, I can feel the sadness overtake me as I contemplate the choice we made. For months we talked about this as an option, but it was so abstract and so easy to talk about when it seemed so far from becoming a reality. Now that we are literally weeks away from doing this, I'm not really sure I'm prepared for this. So many of the things we have done so far have been unseen, and if miracles can happen, will be forgotten if we can pull you through--all the chemo, the tests, the surgeries--these are things that in five years, if we are so lucky, we will have long forgotten about. This however, is so permanent, a constant reminder of the struggles and fears that we will never be able to outrun. If you are one of the lucky ones that gets through this, I can't ever give you that leg back, and as someone whose sole job it is to protect their children, that hurts me so much. I worry that the hydrocephalus has given you learning disabilities; the chemotherapy has given you hearing loss; and now the cancer has claimed your leg, and despite all of this, there is still no guarantee that we can pull you through this. I always said that they could take your leg if they could guarantee that the cancer wouldn't come back in your brain. There's not a doctor on this Earth that could make that statement. So we're faced with doing something so drastic, so life altering, yet I still can't protect you from what lies ahead. Instead I can only make decisions that give you hope, that gives you that one chance. We have to take that chance...

So in a way, the decision is an easy one too. The options for your leg are limited. If they try to remove the tumor and then radiate your leg, there's still a chance that disease will exist and can spread from the leg. Furthermore, if we radiate the leg, we'll have to wait at least a full month before we can start the next round of Ocean Waves, and that gives the disease in other places of your body a chance to wake up once again, and we just can't take that risk. Removing the leg takes disease in that area of out the equation. That leaves only your brain, which is under control right now, as the only area of concern. I'm just not sure there is a way around this decision, and believe me, I've tried to consider everything possible and have tried to negotiate every possible scenario.

I guess it boils down to this, if the decision we made today allows you to be able to read why we had to make this decision, then we know we made the right decision. I hope that one day you can read this and understand why this had to happen to you. That ultimately, it came down to a decision on your life and this was the only way to ensure that your path towards survival had to have one enormous obstacle taken out of your way. I never wished this end for you and would have liked to find any other alternative, but this is the right thing to do for you at this moment in time. Having you with us when you are five, ten, or fifteen will only confirm that what we did was the right thing.

I know every time I write to you I tell you to be brave and be strong, but tonight I need you to share some of that bravery and strength with me because I'm really struggling right now, hoping that we are still giving you a quality of life that allows you to achieve and succeed. There are times when I have my doubts...

Be brave
Be strong
We love you!

Brave Will,

It's been a few days since I last wrote and it's definitely given me time to reflect on where things are headed. Your mom and I are realizing that as saddened as we are by what has to happen to your leg, we simply cannot forget the fact that you are still here and if this leads to recovery, then we know we've done the right thing. I know there are moms and dads who have children with the same disease as you that are in such a tougher spot than you are currently in. I'm sure they would tell us that they would gladly give a leg to save a life if they had the chance. We've not received the news that we ultimately fear the most, and therefore have to still consider ourselves fortunate, as difficult as that is to consider. Even after the surgery has been completed, you are still in a position to fight and survive and that's all we can ever wish for.

I just hope for once that this is it. We continue to be tested and challenged and the decisions on what is "right" are getting harder and harder to come by. I'm not sure how much more your mom and I have left in the tank, and I am certain you probably feel the same way. You've undergone so much in so little time that I just want this to be the final hurdle you have to clear. Please let this be the last difficult decision we have left to make.

For now, we wait. We're holding off on the next round of Ocean Waves until after the surgery, which looks like it will happen on February 12th. Prior to that happening, next week, we're going to give you one last MRI of your brain just to make sure there has been no regression there that would certainly keep us from proceeding with the leg surgery. If that is clear, as we fully expect it to be, then the following week, you'll undergo what is known as a hip disarticulation, which is a fancy way of saying they are going to remove your leg right up to the hip. This is the surest way they have of making sure the disease cannot spread from that area. A number of people have sent us information on other children that have had a similar surgery and we were thrilled to see how they adapted to life many, many years later. And that's the key--if you are able to adapt many, many years later, then the decision was the right one.

Once you recover from surgery, probably about 2 weeks later or so, we'll start the next round of chemo. However, things will change at that point and they'll be able to start giving you much less medicine for two reasons. One, your body simply cannot take any more high dose chemotherapy. Second, once your leg is removed, you will have little, if any, evidence of disease and therefore be moved to a maintenance cycle. To be close to that goal is something that was such a distant thought back in September. To know we are about a month from getting there, gives us all the hope we need to continue.

Your aunt shared with us something she saw on a t-shirt that we will keep in our minds as we go forward with the next steps: Overcome, Improvise, Adapt. We're all going to have to remember those three important words. You will overcome this horrible disease; you will improvise as needed to ensure that your journey through life will not be altered by the handicaps you face; and lastly, you will adapt to whatever challenges stand in your way. And I have some good news for you, little buddy, you won't have to do a single part of any of this by yourself because your mom and dad will be adapting right there with you.

Be brave
Be strong
We love you!

THURSDAY, JANUARY 29, 2009

Brave Will,

It's been a few days and I was just wanted to check in. We continue to enjoy time together at your grandparent's home. We've really been enjoying the amount of time you've been able to spend "tube-free"--no connections to TPN or medicines. It's all felt so normal.

I amazed at how quickly your brothers have adjusted to life with a brother who has special needs. Ben has been so helpful fetching supplies for your mom when you need it and often lays on the floor next to you and talks to you. It's so funny to watch Max every time he approaches you. Whenever he gets within a foot of where you are laying, he stops, backtracks, and cleans his hands with Purell. He doesn't need to be prompted or reminded at all anymore. You're pretty lucky, little man, you've got two awesome older brothers.

I finally got a chance to join your mom at clinic yesterday so I could talk to your doctor about how things are going with you and to ask any questions that have inevitably been building in my mind since we decided to have the surgery. I told her how I just didn't want to lose your leg, and reviewed the options that might be out there for you. What it all boils down to is time, a deadly disease, and an area in your body that is slowly starting to get out of our control. Simply put, if we wait to do this and wait to see if something else could work, we are seriously jeopardizing your life. It's just not something your mom and I can risk. With so many of the decisions that have needed to be made, there was always a "best choice" and a choice that "felt right". Fortunately, up until now, the choice we made fit both descriptions: choosing the chemo plan for you, deciding to send you into surgery even though your counts were gravely low, and so on. This time, however, the choice that "feels right" is to try and save your leg. But it's also clear that this is not the best choice. We've been so aggressive trying to fight this disease that doing anything but amputation is taking a step back and not fighting this as fiercely as we have so far. It's absolutely clear, after spending time with your doctor, that this needs to get done, and done soon. If she had her wish, it would get done tomorrow or the next day, but the earliest it could be coordinated was the 12th. However, if for one minute she feels she is losing control of the disease or that you are in any danger, then she will find a way to push things sooner. That's how serious she views the imminent danger that you have inside of you. We are still planning to take one last peak inside you brain before the surgery to make sure there has been no relapse there. You'll have an MRI Monday morning, and you know by now how I feel about those things. Needless to say, I'm going to enjoy the next three days and try not to think too much about Monday morning.

Before the clinic, we first met with a plastic surgeon to talk about the removal of the affected area on your back. She doesn't feel that plastic surgery will be necessary yet, provided they are able to remove all of the cancerous cells. This should be a pretty easy one to get. The cells appear to be on the surface only, so the removal should not be overly invasive. Once the cells are gone, they will take with it many months of puzzlement, as every doctor that looked at your "birthmark" couldn't figure out what the heck it was. They thought it was many things, but no one thought or feared the worse. Yet it was our first clue for what was to come--we didn't quite know what we were all in for, but that little birthmark came with quite a story that was yet to be told...

Be brave
Be strong
We love you!

SUNDAY, FEBRUARY 01, 2009

Brave Will,

This weekend would definitely be classified as one of those "wake up calls" that you seem to send us every now and again to remind us that we just have to be aware each and every day for things to change, and usually, unfortunately, not for the better. I know that we got ourselves into a little bit of trouble this weekend, and maybe we were able to get out from under it. But the thought never escapes me when something like this happens that maybe, just maybe, one of these times we aren't going to be able to avoid trouble.

Late last week (I think it was Thursday), we began to notice that you had started to eat a lot less, sleep a lot more, and grown increasingly more uncomfortable with the pain from your leg. Even though your mom didn't have to take you to clinic on Friday for a regular appointment, she was concerned about the increasing size of the disease in your leg. When your doctor saw it, she immediately started to make emergency plans for you. That meant taking you back to your ole' stomping grounds on D7, where you were admitted Saturday night.

Today was one of those brutal days where they take lots of pictures of your body and we wait patiently to hear what they found. Today was just your body from your neck down to your thigh. Tomorrow will be your brain, once again. So what were they concerned about? First, why was the leg suddenly larger? Second, had the disease gotten out of control and spread to other areas of your body? Finally, what was causing you to stop eating? They also noticed that your red blood count had plummeted. So the CAT scan was done this afternoon, and fortunately, the doctor didn't see any obvious masses in your body. She again wants to wait for the official reading, and she did want some verification on a couple of areas she was a little unsure of (but didn't believe they were disease related). Your leg, however, has unquestionably grown with disease, and we just don't have the time or ability to control the spread right now. As a result, they have bumped up your surgery from 2/12 to this Tuesday. She simply cannot risk letting the tumors continue to grow and grow for fear that they might go elsewhere in your body.

I guess in some ways, this is a good thing. We don't have to wait in painful anticipation for two more weeks until the surgery was scheduled. Also, after watching things gets worse and worse, there is simply no question in our mind that this step is absolutely necessary for disease control and pain control. If something had turned up in the scan today, we might have thought differently, but as of right now, this is still our best shot for you. We still need to get through the MRI of your brain tomorrow, but provided that goes well, we'll plan on Tuesday being the big surgery day. Of course, it would happen to be on a Tuesday, which always seems to be the days when things happen--your first brain surgery, the day you had breathing problems and we had to sign a DNR, the day your third ventricle failed and they had to put a shunt in despite your gravely low white count. It just seems that these difficult days happen to fall on a Tuesday. The good news is that you have overcome each and every one of those difficult obstacles.

As for those other questions they had today, there's no real answer right now. The doctor does know that you are retaining a lot fluid right now which is causing issues with your appetite and hydration. They are giving you different medicines and nutrition tonight to combat that. At the same time, you are getting a blood transfusion to increase those numbers as well. As your doctor told us today, she wants to wax and buff you so that you are all shiny for the surgery on Tuesday. She needs you to shine when you hit that operating table so that you can be in the best possible physical shape to recover from what you are about to face.

I no longer feel I can apologize for what is going to happen this week. I just know that we have to do this. Looking at the progression of your disease in the leg is your way of telling us that now is the time to do this. You are, and have always, been leading this march. You have had a unique way of letting us know every step of the way what we need to do next, and have done so without uttering a single word. The physical signs on your body, the smiles, the tears, and the cries have all contributed to our ability to give you the right treatment. This certainly would be easier to accomplish if you could just tell us what hurt or where the pain was, but still you have managed to lead us in all the right directions. I have every confidence you will continue to do so as we march onward...

Be brave
Be strong
We love you!

Brave Will,

This is the letter I never thought I would have to write. It's likely going to be one of the hardest and also one of the last that I'll get to do. Today, we hit a major obstacle that you simply cannot overcome this time. There are simply no words that I can possibly come up with to describe the pain that your mom and I are feeling right now. We know you've fought so hard for us for nearly six months and you're body is telling us that you've just had enough.

Today, we found out that the scan that was done yesterday discovered two new tumor locations, one in your stomach and one in your lungs. This might be a result of the tumor in your leg that grew so much that at some point in the last few days it actually broke the femur bone in your leg. It's incomprehensible to me that your condition has deteriorated so much in such a short amount of time. We've gone from being less than 24 hours from you being disease free to now having just days with you in our lives. We are crushed with grief.

When we started this, we knew we were throwing our cards on the table and giving you everything we had in terms of treatment. This gave us our greatest hope, but also meant that we were going for broke and would be left with little options if things went astray. When you take that approach with a disease like the one you have, you simply fight and fight each and every day and pray that your body will respond. We thought we had this thing beat when we saw the tumor in your brain immediately respond. However, that leg never acted the same way and eventually turned on your little body. When your leg broke, the disease broke free and started to take over your tiny, fragile body. Our options at this point are so limited and entirely fruitless. We would only be prolonging the inevitable and at the same, destroying whatever quality time we might have left with you.

I never thought it would end like this. We never saw it coming this way...this fast. I'm devastated at the thought of watching you leave us. While we were overjoyed to hold onto you for six months, it was never going to be enough time, and I just thought we would have you for longer.

My mind is a blur right now and my body and mind appear to be functioning independently. I felt this way in September when we learned of your disease. But the difference then was we had hope--we had a game plan and a chance that things would be different with you. Today, we now know that this simply is not going to be the case--our hope was snatched away in the blink of an eye.

Tonight we sat with your brothers and told them that the doctors just couldn't get rid of all of that cancer in your body and that you would have to go to heaven soon. It was a conversation no parent should ever have with their children. I'm not sure they will completely understand what is happening until it happens. Ben seems uncomfortable talking about it but does realize that soon you will be in heaven looking down upon us. Max was occupied with many other things while we were talking but stopped at one point, stood next to mommy in bed and said "He's too little to go to heaven." It was astounding to hear and we knew all too well how right he is.

I'm not sure where to go from here. I'm not sure how much I need to tell you about what will be happening to you over the next few days, so I may not say much or anything at all. I simply want to cherish however many days we continue to be blessed to have you in our lives until we have to turn you over to those who can free you of this awful disease. Until that happens, we will continue to soak up every second that you spend with us...

Be brave
Be strong
We love you!

THURSDAY, FEBRUARY 05, 2009

Brave Will,

For months we have been asking you to be brave and be strong. So now, when we no longer need you to fight, you are incapable of giving up the battle. It's all you know. From the time you were in your mom's belly, you've been fighting and that has continued for the first six months of your difficult life.

For the last three days, we've done nothing but lay with you and watch you as you've struggled to keep the fight going. Your mom and I have told you time and time again that it's okay for you to go, but it's just not your nature. You are truly a warrior who is going to cherish every moment of your all-too-brief life.

We are at peace knowing that you have been spending your days asleep and without pain. While we miss being able to see those gorgeous eyes, knowing that you are sleeping comfortably, resting up for your next big step is giving us the comfort we need.

We've been so fortunate to have so much support from our friends, family, doctors, and nurses over the past few days. Whenever we feel like we've hit the bottom, there are so many there ready to pull us up and lift our spirits. We'll tell stories about you, about our time here at the hospital, and we start to feel peace once again. The hospital has gone above and beyond to make all of us feel comfortable and supported. One of the doctors even commented that they may have to re-zone the area around your room as a convention center because of the amount of activity. We wouldn't want it any other way...

I've thought a lot about what will happen next, what life will be like and what part you'll play in the rest of our lives. I have no doubt that while Will the person will no longer be with us, your spirit and what you symbolized to so many people in this world in your short, yet powerful life will continue for a very long time. Your story, your spirit, your determination, your courage, and your bravery have inspired so many in so many different ways. It's a legacy I could only dream to leave behind.

Your legacy is complete and solidified, never to be forgotten, so don't feel you need to stick around to make anymore statements and teach yet another lesson. You've provided us with a lifetime of education in such a short amount of time. Feel free now to take a break, relax, and soar...

Be brave
Be strong
We love you!

FRIDAY, FEBRUARY 06, 2009

Brave Will,

Today, at 1:30 PM, you finally soared little buddy, and earned your angel wings. You were, of course, nestled in the arms of your mother and lying right beside Ben and me. Your family and friends surrounded you and boosted you to the heavens. You battled for every breath for nearly twelve hours today--we wouldn't have expected anything less from you.

When you finally took your last breath, your older brother Ben was there by our side to help us deal with our grief. You would have been so proud of him today as he consoled your mom. Only when they took your body away did he finally grasp the full reality of what happened today and was overcome with sadness. But we were glad that he was finally able to ask all of the questions that he had been hiding this whole time.

I know I am at peace with the fact that your soul has finally left your tattered body. However, I never imagined the pain that I would feel knowing you are gone. It's an indescribable emptiness that filled me as I watched you take your last breath. I am so glad to see that you are no longer in pain, no longer affected by this horrible, horrible disease, and no longer fighting an insurmountable battle. But that doesn't make this any easier to handle. I know when your mom and I have some time alone to reflect on the past six months, we will only remember the joy and happiness your short life brought us. But for now we grieve what we lost when you left us today. We are saddened by what could have been and feel cheated at how little time we got to spend with you. It's simply not fair that you were given this fate from the time you were born.

As we were consoled by family members, friends, nurses, doctors, and hospital staff, it was clearly evident that the impact of your life ran very deep in so many people. Lives will be lived differently, for the better, because of how you chose to live your life. You meant so much to so many...

My hope now is to share these letters with your brothers as they get older so they can better understand your life and your legacy. Therefore, I know there are still a couple more left to write. I'm sure there is more to say about your life but the right words to use just escape my weary mind at this time.

Not really sure what to do next. Tonight, we'll deal with the emptiness we are feeling, wake up tomorrow, and try to figure out where to go. When you have spent every minute of every day for the past five months fighting, walking out of the hospital, alone, with nothing left to fight for, has stolen our purpose. But we know there has to be a bigger purpose for this whole ordeal and your mom and I will be desperately digging for what that might be as we struggle through the next days of our life.

Be brave
Be strong
We will always love and never forget you!

(Read at Will's Funeral Service)

Brave Will,

Today, I say goodbye to you for the final time. It's an act I feel like I have rehearsed time and time again since September. I said goodbye to you when we first found out about the horrible disease that had invaded your body. I said goodbye again in September when you awoke on one Tuesday morning and were having so much trouble breathing, the doctors thought that day would be your last. I said goodbye on a Sunday night in September when an operation that had taken place two weeks earlier started to fail and there was very little hope of giving you the relief you needed. I said goodbye on a Tuesday in October when they performed surgery on you even though your body was in no shape to tolerate or recover from it. I said goodbye on a Friday in November when it was thought that the disease had returned with a vengeance in your brain and we were left with no options. I said goodbye last Monday when we knew you had fought your last battle and needed to rest. Finally, I said goodbye last Friday when I watched your last breath escape you and take with it the soul of a beautiful baby that continued to soar above.

Saying goodbye is never an easy thing, but I am able to do it knowing that today is a time for celebration. We celebrate because you are finally at peace, free from a body that failed to match the strength of the heart and soul that lay within. We celebrate today a life that had a greater impact in six short months than many have in a lifetime. We celebrate Brave Will.

Today, I deliver a message to you in front of hundreds of your closest admirers. The message I choose to deliver is not one of pain, anguish, or despair, but rather one of peace and acceptance. While your mom and I are sad that you are gone and sad that we won't be able to hold your little hand, kiss your chubby cheeks or lay our hands upon your bald head, we choose not to mourn your passing and grieve our loss. Cancer has done too much to our family in such a short amount of time—we cannot let it continue to devastate us. Instead, we need to show this disease who really won the battle in the end.

Your mom and I have talked about how your life was like an intermission of our own lives. We can't associate you with our time in Wilton because you were born after we moved. And we can't connect you to our new home in Ballston Lake because we haven't yet moved in. So instead, our time with you filled that nice little gap of time that we were left without an identity. But an intermission is fleeting, temporary, and passing. You life was none of these things. Your life was profound, inspirational, and courageous. Your actions and legacy will allow us to continue to let you live in our hearts well beyond the next phase of our life, and the one after that, and the one after that. An intermission, my little friend, has a distinct beginning and an end. What you have left behind has no apparent length of time and no clear conclusion.

I admit, however, that there have been times over the past few days that I have viewed your life as a tease. I feel cheated from a life that I will never get to see grow. I wonder who you would have grown to look like. I wonder whether you would have taken on the quiet, thoughtfulness of your brother Ben or would have been fearless and outgoing like your brother Max. I think about what might have been and it saddens me. Like any parent, whenever a new child is brought into this world, I couldn't help but to have grand plans in my mind. Plans for our family, plans for my three sons, and plans for you and me. It hurts not to be able to see those dreams come true. But to view your life as tease would be a selfish and neglectful act. It would fail to recognize what you have accomplished in your short life and will continue to accomplish from up above.

I also struggle with the "what happens next" phase of our life. I think about the next few days, weeks, and months, and know they will be incredibly challenging. I hope that this is the hardest thing that we will ever have to go through as a family, as I am not sure that the strength and courage you have displayed will be there for us should we encounter another crisis. I know life will go on at some point, but I think it might be easier for me. I worry about your mom and how she'll manage her life without you. You see, buddy, there isn't anyone out there that I know who has wanted to be a mommy more than your mom. Like a doctor or a fireman who was called to his or her profession, your mom was meant to be a mom. And boy, is she good at it. I'm glad she'll still have two boys to look after and be challenged by, but I know she'll always have a void that I just won't be able to fill. For the last six months, her life was you. For 24 hours a day, seven days a week, she was completely devoted to your well being. It's all she has known. Her life has been hospitals, MRIs, chemotherapy, line flushes, TPN, and clinic. But more importantly, her life has been about Will Hladun. I take solace in the fact that because of her devotion to you, she will never let your memory go and her next mountain to climb will be to ensure that your name lives on in the lives of the thousands that you have touched.

I think back to when we found out about your diagnosis and about how bleak the outlook was. You were two months old at the time and I wondered, out loud at times, if it would be better to have you go then versus having more time with you, if we were still going to lose you in the end. Would more time with you make the inevitable final outcome only that much harder? I really struggled with that for days. But as I look back on the past five months of our life, I am eternally grateful for every second that I had you in my life. I'm grateful for the first smile, the first coo, and the first giggle. I never thought I would get to see any of those things when this all first started.

I am amazed, in reflection, that the battle only lasted five months. If you had told me that it had been only five months from the time you were diagnosed, I would not have believed it. The days just seemed to go by invisibly, blending from one to the next. Your mom and I chose to focus not on what the day and time was, but more on how we spent that time. As a result, those five months felt more like five years. The time we spent with you allowed us to feel something very special that we weren't sure we would feel if we lost you and that's this: We have not one single regret regarding your life, your care, or your treatment. We know we did everything we could to keep you in our lives, but still give you a quality of life you so greatly deserved. We know we made decisions that took into account your well being but also gave us the hope we needed to continue. And in the end, when it was clear that our options were limited, we let you make the final decision to go quietly and peacefully.

Your mom always said you were an old soul. That when you blinked your eyes at us, they seemed to be telling us a story not from the eyes of a infant, but rather someone who appeared to know so much more and had a wisdom that was unlike any other. We just knew last week that you were telling us it was time. We fought and fought for so long, we knew you were tired and needed to stop. When we decided to cease treatment, you quickly drifted off to sleep and stayed sleeping for five long days. You didn't struggle and you weren't in pain—a gift to us that we will never forget. You just slept and we grew more peaceful.

As I stood there yesterday at your celebration and shook hands, hugged and kissed hundreds of your greatest admirers, I was overcome with a feeling of pride. As a father, I can't think of single greater emotion than wanting to be proud of your son or daughter. The words I heard about being a better parent, a better citizen, a better person. The words I heard about living life differently and changing ways. That's what you were able to accomplish in six short months. I am honored that I got to share your story with so many around the world. You were too special for just your mom and me to hold on to—you left the world a better place than you found it. I can only hope, in my long life, to accomplish a small fraction of what you did in your short life.

I am so proud of you, my little friend.

Be brave
Be strong
We will always love and never forget you!

Acknowledgments

Over the course of our journey with Will, the amount of support and guidance we received was endless. We simply would not have been able to bear one single day without the help of so many. It is impossible to thank everyone who supported us through actions or words. However, there are a few that we want to specifically recognize. We will never be able to say the right words and find a way to repay the generosity, but please know how highly we regard each and every one of you:

Our parents, sisters, brothers-in law, aunts, uncles, cousins, nieces, and nephews

Ben and Darcy Shaw, Will's Godparents

Dr. Joanne Porter

Dr. Jennifer Cerone

Dr. Bill Fredette

Father Kenneth Gregory

The amazing nurses at Albany Medical Center

Management and staff at Hilton Garden Inn Albany Medical Center

BBL Development Group

Staff at Queensbury Union Free School District

Log Jam Restaurant

D'Andrea's Liquor

Trios Pizzeria and Delicatessen

Ashley Brown Photography

Studio D

Pediatric Dentistry of Glens Falls

Leah Dwornik Photography

Hayes Paving

DA Collins

Tech Electric

Volpe Custom Homes

Genieve's Home and Garden Decor

Salvadore Funeral Home

> …and to our closest friends, our endless supporters, and thousands of others who visited, donated, and offered us words of kindness and hope.